Therapeutically Applied Role-Playing Games

Therapeutically Applied Role-Playing Games provides a comprehensive approach to implementing therapeutically applied role-playing game (TA-RPG) groups for mental health practitioners.

When facilitated by a trained professional, TA-RPGs are a powerful tool for insight, growth, and change for individuals and communities. The Game to Grow Method of Therapeutically Applied Role-Playing Games is a transdiagnostic, transtheoretical, group intervention developed over a decade of practice using Dungeons & Dragons and other popular tabletop role-playing game systems, as well as leveraging therapeutic factors from acceptance and commitment therapy, marriage and family therapy, drama therapy, and interpersonal process groups. TA-RPGs are conceptualized as a gaming system layered on top of established intervention techniques. They can accommodate a multitude of game systems and align with theoretical mechanisms for change found across therapeutic orientations.

This work serves as a comprehensive training manual for TA-RPGs, providing a valuable resource for mental health professionals interested in incorporating TA-RPGs into their practice.

Elizabeth D. Kilmer, PhD, is a clinical psychologist with ADHD and the Director of Education and training with Game to Grow. Her work focuses on the use of applied games with diverse populations.

Adam D. Davis, MAEd, is a co-founder and co-executive director of Game to Grow. His career has focused on using innovative ways to help people learn, connect, and grow.

Jared N. Kilmer, PhD, is an autistic clinical psychologist and the Director of Counseling Services of Game to Grow. His career focuses on the utilization of TA-RPGs among military veteran and neurodiverse children and adolescents.

Adam R. Johns, MA, LMFT, is a co-founder and co-executive director of Game to Grow. He has dedicated his career to the improved understanding of the ways in which games can positively impact our lives.

Therapeutically Applied Role-Playing Games

The Game to Grow Method

By Elizabeth D. Kilmer,
Adam D. Davis, Jared N. Kilmer,
and Adam R. Johns

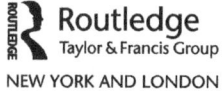

Routledge
Taylor & Francis Group

NEW YORK AND LONDON

First published 2023
by Routledge
605 Third Avenue, New York, NY 10158

and by Routledge
4 Park Square, Milton Park, Abingdon, Oxon, OX14 4RN

Routledge is an imprint of the Taylor & Francis Group, an informa business

ISBN: 978-1-032-25187-5 (hbk)
ISBN: 978-1-032-25185-1 (pbk)
ISBN: 978-1-003-28196-2 (ebk)

DOI: 10.4324/9781003281962

Typeset in New Baskerville
by Apex CoVantage, LLC

To everyone who ever created a story, and found themselves inside of it.

Contents

Foreword

Raffael Boccamazzo, PsyD

This book is more than a decade in the making. I cannot wait for people to read it and be as inspired by it as much as I am by its authors. Before I sing its praises, a bit of story and reminiscence:

In spring 2011, while I drove to my doctoral training site working with children and adolescents, I had a moment of inspiration: tabletop role-playing games (TTRPGs) like *Dungeons & Dragons* as a vehicle for thera-peutic interventions! After all, role-playing has a long, rich history as an intervention across multiple schools of psychology and psychiatry, in addition to play therapy, psychodrama, and drama therapy as standalone concepts, and using games as a method of teaching is widely accepted by teachers and workshop trainers across multitudes of disciplines. This was a natural combination! As an aside, I eventually learned of other overlaps such as science fiction writer H.G. Wells' influence on both the development of play therapy through his book *Floor Games* (Mitchell & Friedman, 1994) and *Dungeons & Dragons* through his game *Little Wars* (Peterson, 2012).

Self-assured of my utter brilliance in birthing a genius idea absolutely no one else had ever thought of in the history of time or the vast expanse of the universe, I excitedly called a friend of mine in my doctoral pro-gram who had similar, nerdy interests, and I shared my 100% original, unique, never-before-conceived idea with her, waiting for her to marvel at its genesis. As soon as I said "*Dungeons & Dragons* as a therapeutic inter-vention!" she went silent, and after a moment asked, "Who told you?"

"What?" I responded.

"Who told you we're doing that?" she asked me in the most suspicious tone I had ever heard from her.

"Wait. You're doing that at your training site?!"

Two things were suddenly clear to me: (1) I was not as original as I thought—a lesson which would be repeated many times in my career—and (2) I needed to know more.

She proceeded to tell me of a student at her site using TTRPGs as a way of deliberately helping adolescents practice interpersonal skills. It was already being done! My idea might not have been original, but the validation energized me to put together a pitch on TTRPG-based group therapy for my training site that year! It was a few years later that I learned it was two of this book's authors—Adam D. Davis and Adam R. Johns ("the Adams")—who were the ones running the groups at my friend's training site, with Adam D. Davis beginning in 2011 and Adam R. Johns beginning in 2012.

I later met the Adams while I was running my own TTRPG groups for a local agency—coincidentally the one at which they started. We eventually co-participated on panels about TA-RPGs and got to know each other better. There was something that immediately struck me about them; they had a remarkable ability to connect with people and to connect people to each other. It was because of this ability and their prolific public advocacy work that other practitioners and students, both nationally and internationally, started saying, "Hey! I'm doing this too, and I thought I was the only one!" or "This is amazing! I want to do this!" The interest was there. The love of TTRPGs was there. Yet people were largely operating and creating in isolation, unaware of the growing movement to legitimize TTRPGs in learning and clinical spaces.

The Adams started to connect the dots to other people prominently incorporating TTRPGs in their practices and work. This included, among others, Hawke Robinson—a recreational therapist who had been using TTRPGs in his practice in Washington State for years; Jack Berkenstock Jr., MHS in Pennsylvania whose work with incarcerated youth incorporating TTRPGs evolved into a successful nonprofit group; Megan Connell, PsyD, ABPP in North Carolina—a psychologist who does amazing work using TTRPGs with adolescent girls; Sarah Lynn Bowman, PhD—a game scholar in Texas whose books focused on the transformative power of TTRPGs; and eventually Elizabeth and Jared N. Kilmer—the other authors of this book, and students at the time—who were doing utterly fascinating work using TTRPGs to help veterans with posttraumatic stress disorder within the US Department of Veterans Affairs in Texas. It turned out that the Kilmers shared the Adams' love of teaching people about the power of TTRPGs and their passion for building community.

Over the ensuing years, many of the folks listed earlier have become colleagues and friends. We have had countless, robust conversations (and even debates) about how to best develop and promote TTRPGs in clinical and learning settings. Many of us have developed our own trainings and theories. Throughout those conversations at that time, both the Adams and the Kilmers never ceased to amaze me with the utter diversity of ideas they both brought to their shared theories, as well as the diversity of ideas they invited.

This book is rooted in the four authors' collective experiences, inter-ests, and a shared desire to promote TTRPGs as a vibrant, accessible, and ultimately fun way of helping people find fulfillment and joy in their lives. Between them, the authors bring expertise in cognitive behavioral therapy, acceptance commitment therapy, drama therapy, marriage and family therapies, trauma therapy, pedagogical theories, and experience serving the diverse populations of all ages with whom they have worked. This includes serving their clients in a refreshingly neurodiversity-affirming manner—a present rarity, from the perspective of this autistic and ADHD psychologist.

This book is a result of their collective joy in the topic of TTRPGs, their effort to build up the knowledge and appreciation of the power of play in clinical and learning settings, and their infectious enthusiasm to serve their clients and build community. They often repeat the idiom, "A rising tide raises all boats."

This book raises the tide.

Raffael Boccamazzo, PsyD
Clinical Director—Take This, Inc.

Mitchell, R. R., & Friedman, H. S. (1994). *Sandplay: Past, present and future*. Routledge.

Peterson, J. (2012). *Playing at the world: A history of simulating wars, people and fantastic adventures, from chess to role-playing games*. Unreason Press.

Acknowledgments

Jared—you introduced me to tabletop role-playing games, and have been with me every step of the way since. I wouldn't be here without those Sunday afternoons spent playing together. Mom, Dad, Stephanie, and Andrew—you taught me I could do whatever I wanted when I grew up and you continue to encourage me when I get stuck. Jennifer—you helped me gain the confidence and knowledge to achieve my most intimidating goals. Katrina—you provided me with an opportunity to start my very first TA-RPG group and worked with me to see it flourish. Amee—your championship, support, and advice has been instrumental as I've grown in this field. And Badger—you barked at me when I worked too long, and have been my constant companion through this writing process.

—Elizabeth D. Kilmer

Kristen, my lighthouse. Your unwavering support makes *everything* possible. Louise, your snores while sleeping on my chest provided a soundtrack to so much of this book. Margaret, you saw something unique in my misfit style and gave me a chance to show it. Patti and Lee, you sat me down and told me I was on to something big. Jason, you pointed me toward my future in both drama therapy and RPGs. Wes, you gave the pep talk that kept us going. Finally, Adam 2.0, thanks for your companionship in uncharted lands, for the whiteboard brainstorms and the shabu shabu, and for the very particular set of skills you acquired over a very long career.

—Adam D. Davis

I would like to thank the following people for their support and influence upon the person I've become:

To my academic mentor, Dr. Camilo Ruggero, for teaching me to think and write critically. To my former supervisors, Drs. Susan Matlock-Hetzel, Melissa Switzer, and Meredith Shaw for supporting, encouraging, and shaping my crazy ideas. To my wife and colleagues for putting up with my persnickety opinions. To the veteran who once exclaimed, "F*ck CBT! D&D is for me!" You know who you are. To my family and friends for all the cheerleading. It kept me going.

—Jared N. Kilmer

To Allysa and Sabriel, without whom I would have lost motivation long ago. You are forever my inspiration, my roots, and my fuel. You keep me grounded all while helping me reach for the stars above me. I owe you all I am, and more. To my brothers Alex and Ben, who continue to amaze me with their brilliance and kindness. To my father, David, and my mother, Helene, who taught me to dream and never give up. To my friends Zach, Elizabeth, and Xella, who can make me laugh even on the hardest days of my life. Finally, to Adam Prime, who has never left my side in the long journey that I have undertaken, in the face of both feast and famine. You will always be my partner and my friend, no matter what paths we may travel.

—Adam R. Johns

An Introduction to Therapeutically Applied Role-Playing Games

Therapeutically Applied Role-Playing Games (TA-RPGs) are an approach to group treatment that catalyze the inherent benefits of collaborative storytelling games with established group intervention methods. This book will cover the Game to Grow Method of TA-RPGs, though it is important to note there are multiple approaches to TA-RPGs (i.e., Berkenstock, 2021; Boccamazzo & Connell, 2019; Connell et al., 2020). This intervention was originally developed to use the Dungeons & Dragons tabletop role-playing game (TTRPG) system to help participants become more confident, creative, and socially capable through the intentional leveraging of therapeutic factors from drama therapy, interpersonal process group therapy, cognitive behavioral therapies, and DIR/Floortime approaches. However, TA-RPGs can accommodate a multitude of game systems and theoretical mechanisms for change found in various therapeutic orientations. The flexibility of the approach allows for TA-RPGs to be applied across multiple settings (e.g., community mental health, residential mental health treatment, school settings, and community settings) and populations. These groups fall into two broad categories, differentiated by the goals and populations of the groups: social flourishing groups and counseling groups.

TA-RPGs are conceptualized as a gaming system layered on top of established group interventions. In this way, role-playing games (RPGs) become the vector for delivering a therapeutic intervention, as opposed to the intervention itself. As such, strong training in group interventions is vital. The game is a pathway by which traditional therapeutic mechanisms of change are utilized and enhanced.

As with other group therapy interventions, TA-RPGs can provide a more efficient delivery of treatment through the ability of a single provider to treat multiple clients at once. Group interventions have been found to be appropriate for a wide range of diagnoses and populations (Blackmore et al., 2012, Burlingame et al., 2003, Philipsen et al., 2007, Tillitski, 1990, Wergeland et al., 2014). Additionally, interventions in a group setting can take advantage of therapeutic group interaction phenomena. For example, many process groups rely on therapeutic

DOI: 10.4324/9781003281962-1

factors such as the social microcosm, altruism, and universality, which are absent, or considerably less present, in individual therapy (Yalom & Leszcz, 2020). TA-RPGs are intentionally delivered in a group format to take advantage of the inherent benefits found in both group psychotherapy and collaborative multiplayer games.

The History of Game to Grow and the Game to Grow Method of Therapeutically Applied Role-Playing Games

Game to Grow is a 501(c)(3) nonprofit organization dedicated to the use of games of all kinds for therapeutic, educational, and community growth. Adam D. Davis, MA Ed, and Adam R. Johns, MA, LMFT, are the co-founders and co-executive directors of Game to Grow, Elizabeth D. Kilmer, PhD, is the Director of Education and Training, and Jared N. Kilmer, PhD, is the Director of Counseling services. Together, Dr. Jared N. Kilmer, Dr. Elizabeth D. Kilmer, Adam D. Davis, and Adam R. Johns have helped raise the profile of TA-RPGs into the professional practices and lives of people around the world. Through direct services, training programs, the game Critical Core, and talks at conventions around the world, these four individuals have had a significant and undeniable impact on the field of therapeutically applied games.

Johns and Davis met in graduate school in 2011, where they began to use TTRPGs as a way to promote social growth and improvement for neurodiverse teens. Davis was working as a social group facilitator for neurodiverse teens, and invited Johns to join him as a co-facilitator. The group used TTRPGs, like Dungeons & Dragons (D&D), as a fun activity to help participants connect with each other. It worked well, as the group participants found the game engaging and the collaborative stories compelling.

Davis and Johns began to use the concepts from drama therapy and couple and family therapy that they were learning in graduate school, as well as Davis' years in participatory theater and experiential education, to inform their use of D&D as an intentional tool for growth. The participants that they saw in those games began to grow and improve in profound ways, sometimes from the progression of the story, the growth of their own characters, or the experiences that they had at the table as a player. Not only that, but participants were excited and encouraged to return to the group each week due to the fun and engagement of the game. Participants, who would often require their parents to incentivize their attendance at school or participation in therapy, would finish their homework early to ensure that they could attend their weekly TTRPG social skills group (as they were called at the time). One parent described it as her son "eating his vegetables without knowing he was eating his vegetables."

After seeing how effective TTRPGs could be as a tool for personal growth, especially when facilitated intentionally, Johns and Davis founded a company called Wheelhouse Workshop, LLC. As it grew in popularity within the Seattle area, Adam R. Johns and Adam D. Davis traveled around the United States to speak at conventions and present at professional conferences about their unique treatment approach and the tremendous growth that they were seeing in their participants. Presenting at professional conferences and academic institutions prompted a concretization of the methodology. What had existed only in practice and jotted into notebooks was flushed out and presented to hundreds of therapists and other professionals. Many of the talks at conventions were focused on inspirational stories from the burgeoning field of "intentional gaming," and were so well received that Adam R. Johns and Adam D. Davis began to be known as "The Adams."

Audiences around the world found the therapeutic application of games to be inspiring. Touched by tales of success and growth, many commented on the similarities between Davis and Johns' stories and their own personal journeys involving TTRPGs. Additionally, Johns and Davis learned that they were not the only professionals who had recognized the connection between TTRPGs and personal growth. They met many individuals already doing similar work in their own varied fields. This brought about a shared feeling of excitement and validation that others had come to similar conclusions about the therapeutic potential of TTRPGs. Through these conventions and presentations, Johns and Davis made many personal connections with prominent individuals in the field of applied RPGs (i.e., Dr. Virginia Spielmann, Dr. Raffael Boccamazzo, Dr. Megan Connell, Hawke Robinson, and Jack Berkenstock), and inspired others to pursue careers in the therapeutic application of games. They were beginning to expand the field of TA-RPGs, though they would not know the impact of those early talks until years later.

Some of those connections included professionals who were so passionate and excited about the concept of TA-RPGs that a collaboration of ideas and approaches was inevitable. One of those important early connections, made in 2016, was Dr. Virginia Spielmann, PhD, OTR/L, who was working on the development of a TA-RPG called Critical Core. Davis and Johns found that Dr. Spielmann's approaches and perspectives from occupational therapy and DIR/Floortime therapy leveraged many similar concepts to the ones being used by Johns and Davis, but under different names. This synergy of ideas would come up again and again in the development of this model. Virginia contributed important concepts from the International Council on Development and Learning (ICDL) and DIR/Floortime into the design of Critical Core and played an important role in shaping the Core Capacities described in this book.

Another undeniably important connection made during this time occurred while presenting at the Penny Arcade Expo South in 2016. Dr. Jared N. Kilmer and Dr. Elizabeth D. Kilmer, in seeing their first presentation from "the Adams," found the ideas to be in line with their own experiences of games and psychology, inspiring them to dive into independent research and practice of TA-RPGs. They began to develop their own methodology by utilizing relational and cognitive behavioral approaches, such as Acceptance and Commitment Therapy (ACT), Dialectical Behavior Therapy (DBT), and interpersonal process group theory. They were particularly excited to explore applications of their model for their populations of interest, including individuals who have experienced trauma, substance use disorder, severe mental illness, and neurodivergence. Later that year, Jared began a group for veterans in residential posttraumatic stress disorder (PTSD) treatment at the Doris Miller Department of Veterans Affairs Medical Center in Waco, Texas, as well as in an outpatient psychosocial rehabilitation and recovery center for individuals with severe mental illness. Though some staff and veterans were initially skeptical of this play-based intervention, the feedback from group participants quickly turned the tide among hospital staff and patients alike. Veterans praised the groups for the insight, confidence, and camaraderie gained, with one veteran describing the intervention as "the only thing that has ever really helped." The group was so popular that when Jared moved to the Dallas VA Medical Center, he was asked to train staff to keep current groups running. While at the Dallas VA, Jared founded TA-RPG groups in residential substance use, homeless domiciliary, and psychosocial rehabilitation clinics.

Over the course of several years Jared, Elizabeth, Adam, and Adam continued to connect, sharing stories, experiences, and excitement around the power and potential growth of the TA-RPG field. This relationship, and these experiences, would ultimately shape the model and approach in this text. In many ways, the foundations of this approach would not have been possible without the excitement and shared enthusiasm of geek and gaming culture.

In 2017, Adam R. Johns and Adam D. Davis co-founded Game to Grow, along with founding board members, Dr. Kirk Honda, Erick Blandin, and Aurora Newcomb. The Adams were confident in the methods they had been using and the impact of their work, but knew it would take more than just the two of them to significantly expand that impact beyond Seattle. Game to Grow was founded to be more than just an organization doing good, but a platform for a powerful message: Games have incredible power to improve lives, and that potential can be maximized when games are facilitated by a trained professional. From there, with the help of an establishing grant from Child's Play Charity, Johns and Davis were able to focus on expanding the services and mission of Game to Grow far beyond the work that had been done by Wheelhouse

Workshop. The vision was clear: a game in every clinic, a game in every school, and a game in every hospital.

In 2018, Elizabeth D. Kilmer started her first TA-RPG group at the Dallas Children's Advocacy Center for adolescents who had experienced trauma. This group quickly grew in popularity, resulting in the opportunity for Elizabeth to collaborate with and train several co-facilitators to continue her groups. Following her work at the Children's Advocacy Center, Elizabeth had her own opportunity to run a TA-RPG group at the Dallas VA. A testament to their early commitment to supporting growth in this field, many of the groups the Kilmers started are still running today, thanks to the clinicians they trained in their methodology.

Having completed the transition to Game to Grow, Adam R. Johns and Adam D. Davis began to bring on more team members to serve a wider population within the Seattle area. Johns and Davis distilled their methodology into didactic instructions in order to communicate it to other facilitators eager to learn their unique approach to social flourishing. In 2019, Game to Grow launched a Kickstarter campaign for Critical Core, a simplified TTRPG starter set designed to cultivate social confidence among neurodiverse youth. The demand was strong and it was fully funded within eight hours. Between training new Game to Grow facilitators, and the development of Critical Core, Johns and Davis built a crucial understanding of how to teach their successful approach to others.

Concurrently, in 2019, Drs. Jared N. Kilmer and Elizabeth D. Kilmer moved to Washington State where Elizabeth founded a TA-RPG group with the primary care clinic at the American Lake VA, prior to the two officially joining the Game to Grow team. With the Kilmers' training in clinical psychology and background in research, as well as their own unique knowledge and approaches to TA-RPGs, they collaborated with Johns and Davis to build a solid and comprehensive foundation for TA-RPGs to support social flourishing.

In 2022, after several years of further writing and development, including design work by Gavin Cheng and concept collaboration with Dr. Virginia Spielmann, the Critical Core box set was released, providing an opportunity to introduce teachers, therapists, educators, and like-minded individuals to TA-RPGs. Coupled with Game to Grow's comprehensive training program, those eager to fold TA-RPGs into their professional practices gained access to the tools and resources necessary to engage in this rewarding work.

Over years together, Adam D. Davis, Adam R. Johns, Elizabeth D. Kilmer, and Jared N. Kilmer have combined their passion, their experiences, and their knowledge to collaborate on this text with one goal in mind: to bring the power of therapeutically applied games into more people's lives. This text represents the many hours of impassioned discussion, argument, and personal growth, finally brought into a cohesive and comprehensive text to help others join us in this field together.

Introduction to Tabletop Role-Playing Games

RPGs describe a broad category of games that can range from highly active and social experiences, such as live action role playing (LARP), to minimally active and solitary experiences, such as many video game RPGs. A TTRPG is a style of RPG that typically takes place around a table, or comparable virtual environment, and occurs in the presence of other people. TTRPGs are collaborative storytelling games and typically consist of a game master (GM), who describes the story's world and arbitrates rules, alongside several players, each of whom is responsible for role-playing their own character within the story. The GM takes the role of lead storyteller and referee, narrating and sharing information about the places, creatures, and people that make up the setting of the adventure. As players determine and describe how their characters interact with the story elements outlined by the GM, their characters' actions are determined to succeed or fail on the basis of the game's formal set of rules and game mechanics (referred to as the "game system"). Because these systems are designed to determine outcomes for an infinitely varied set of actions, players are afforded opportunities to be creative, improvise, and affect the direction and outcome of the narrative. Players work together to solve puzzles, engage in combat, and hunt for treasure and knowledge. While each TTRPG game system provides a jumping off point for rules, adventures, and fantasy worlds in which to set these adventures, it is common practice for individuals leading and playing the game to develop their own "house rules" and stories.

Many TTRPGs have accessory items designed to enhance the gaming experience, such as digital or physical maps, miniatures to represent characters, specialized dice, and even miniature sets. Though these items are not required for gameplay, the creation of and engagement with these items can serve as a secondary hobby. Further, they can be an additional source of potential community. Players who enjoy collecting dice or painting miniatures have an added source of shared enjoyment and opportunities for connection with others who share these adjunctive hobbies.

For a more in-depth breakdown of TTRPGs, the terminology used in the hobby, refer to Chapter 2.

Why Tabletop Role-Playing Games?

TTRPGs provide a valuable avenue to social connection and a framework to support the development of social skills. Social connection and wellness are reciprocally linked, forming a feedback loop. Diminished positive social connections is a significant risk factor for mental health diagnoses, and those impacted by such diagnoses are at increased risk of becoming socially isolated (Chou et al., 2011; Eussen et al., 2013; Orsmond et al., 2013). As a consequence of social isolation, an individual's ability to connect and communicate with others may be underdeveloped or atrophy over time, ultimately resulting in an over-reliance on medical professionals and additional resources to assist in addressing one's concerns. Indeed, maladaptive social skills and isolation are themselves symptoms of several mental health diagnoses such as depression, anxiety, autism spectrum disorder (ASD), and posttraumatic stress disorder (PTSD; Frueh et al., 2001; Segrin & Flora, 2000). Further, the perception of reduced social connectedness is associated with increased mortality and morbidity risk (Cacioppo & Cacioppo, 2014; Umberson & Karas Montez, 2010). In contrast, increasing social efficacy and connectedness has been linked to better mental health outcomes (Tew et al., 2012). In a study examining PTSD symptoms and psychological growth after trauma, veterans with higher social connectedness reported higher levels of growth following traumatic events (Tsai et al., 2015). Likewise, research on outcomes following residential treatment for substance use found that individuals with stronger social networks had better mental health and sobriety outcomes (Warren et al., 2007).

Special Note

The Game to Grow Method was designed to empower individuals who need support in the domain of interpersonal connectedness. While the youth and adults who access Game to Grow services are often diagnosed with a neurodivergence, have experienced trauma, or both, we do not believe that every neurodivergent individual needs to learn social skills, nor do we believe that to be neurodivergent is to be inherently flawed.

Because space in this text is limited, we do not spell this out each time we discuss different populations, diagnostic criteria, common social challenges, and related research findings. Throughout, our priority was to clearly outline our approach. This method is an alternative to skill-based training programs that choose to use external controls and "rules" to shape behaviors, often disregarding the complex internal lives of the individuals being served. It is for individuals in distress, who lack social confidence, who struggle with self-advocacy, and who have not been supported to discover who they want to be and how they want to socially interact with the often exclusionary and unforgiving world around them.

As you read, remember that not all neurodivergent individuals are disordered, nor do they need to be cured of their divergent ways of experiencing the world. The world is enhanced for everyone when we celebrate the rich tapestry of the human experience, and it would be better still if we could all learn to laugh, play, and grow together.

Though the definition of "social skills" varies across the literature, "social skills" typically refers to a constellation of abilities that support an individual in successfully navigating social situations to achieve predictable outcomes. This constellation of abilities can include competencies in perspective taking, collaboration, verbal and nonverbal communication, and emotional and behavioral regulation. In children, underdeveloped social skills have been consistently linked with problems in school, as well as emotional and behavioral difficulties (Cook et al., 2008; Gifford-Smith & Brownell, 2003). In comparison, strong social skills have been associated with measures of individual resilience and academic achievement in children and adolescents (Rajendran & Videka, 2006). The strength of social-emotional skills in early elementary school has been found to be positively correlated with educational, employment, and mental health outcomes over a decade later (Jones et al., 2015). Strong social skills and social networks convey positive benefits across children, adolescents, and adults, which suggest that interventions targeting an individual's ability to interact and connect with others are likely to be beneficial across the lifespan. Interventions targeting social skills have been found to be effective in improving quality of life outcomes with individuals with mental health disorders (e.g., depression, schizophrenia, ASD; Kasari et al., 2012; Cuijpers et al., 2008; Mueser & Bellack, 2009).

Notably, traditional social skills training, often delivered in clinic settings, may be less effective than interventions that allow flexible practice with real peers (Mikami et al., 2017). Further, traditional social skills training programs have been criticized for an overreliance on teaching social rules in a vacuum—without the contextual nuances of the real-world social milieu (Bottema-Beutel et al., 2018). In fact, traditional social skills training with autistic youth can improve participant's knowledge of social skills without affecting the enactment of such skills (Gates et al., 2017).

In contrast to traditional social skills groups, TTRPGs can create opportunities for social learning with peers in a low-risk setting. Autistic youth who participated in TTRPG groups reported higher scores on a quality-of-life index following participation in the groups, particularly in the areas of friendships and emotional well-being (Kato, 2019). In addition to social competence, participation in TTRPG groups has been linked with a host of positive outcomes, from increased creativity, to positive attitude changes, to better moral reasoning. In a study that explored verbally mediated creativity in TTRPG players, electronic RPG players, and non-players, the TTRPG players performed higher across measures, especially in areas of flexibility, fluency, and uniqueness (Chung, 2012). TTRPG play is not only correlated with higher creativity. It may, in fact, be able to improve participant creativity. Another study found that participants who engaged in a TTRPG group for four weeks had significant improvements in measures of cognitive creativity compared to a control group who did not play TTRPGs (Dyson et al., 2016). Researcher-participants who engaged in a TTRPG with the express intention of facilitating personal growth (described as a "transformative role-playing game") found their experience with TTRPGs supported team building, self-exploration, and collaborative creativity (Daniau, 2016). Additionally, role-playing may be able to influence stronger attitude changes than observation. This was demonstrated in a study where smokers were asked to role-play a persuasive argument against smoking or simply observe the persuasive argument (Elms, 1966). Similarly, RPGs may be able to support the development of critical ethical reasoning skills in participants through experiences in gameplay (Simkins & Steinkuehler, 2008). After participating in TTRPG encounters specifically designed to support collaborative decision-making around ethical quandaries, participants demonstrated growth on moral development in comparison to participants in a control group (Wright et al., 2017).

Therapeutically Applied Role-Playing Games

In addition to the benefits identified in playing TTRPGs recreationally with peers, there is a growing body of research on the efficacy of TA-RPGs (Arenas et al., 2022; Henrich & Worthington, 2021). TA-RPGs utilize established therapeutic techniques in concert with the TTRPG framework to support participant growth. For example, this body of research builds on the established knowledge of the utility of role-play in therapy (Kipper & Ritchie, 2003), as well as that of simulation training (Low et al., 2020; Okuda, 2008; Joyner & Young, 2006). Research across several settings and populations has identified potential benefits of the use of TA-RPGs with children, adolescents, and adults.

One of the earliest academic papers that specifically discusses potential utility of TTRPGs in therapy was a case study where a therapist utilized D&D as a way to connect with their client. When this therapist experienced difficulty establishing rapport with a client with a diagnosis of schizoid personality disorder, the therapist utilized conversations about D&D to build rapport and support the therapy process (Blackmon, 1994). Since this paper, more research on the intentional use of TTRPGs in group therapeutic settings have emerged. For example, quality improvement projects across multiple VA settings have found increases in investment in and adherence to treatment, attendance, creativity, playfulness, frustration tolerance, self-esteem, confidence, humor, forgiveness, connection to others, empathy, and well-being, as well as reduced impulsivity and depressive symptoms (Kilmer, 2020; Kilmer & Kilmer, 2018; Roy, 2019; Battles et al., 2021). In a TA-RPG group for adults with social anxiety, participants reported increased social confidence, and reported the skills they practiced in the game translated into their real lives (Abbott et al., 2021). TA-RPGs have also been used to support the social emotional development of a group of gifted adolescents (Rosselet & Stauffer, 2013).

The TA-RPG Experience

Much of the therapeutic growth in TA-RPGs is covert, and not inherently perceived as "therapy." Individuals engaged in TA-RPG groups have described them as "exciting," "inspiring," and "a respite from traditional therapy processes and the stress of [their] daily life" (Kilmer & Kilmer, 2018). The role-playing environment is of low risk compared to reality, and players can be encouraged to try out solutions without fear of real-world consequences.

A well-run TTRPG is a collaborative and enriching process between GM and players, and TA-RPG groups are no different. TTRPGs offer novel and narratively rich gameplay experiences. As intended storylines determine only a fraction of the gameplay, it is the players around the table that drive the story in a particular direction and determine the overall experience. During TA-RPG sessions, participants are guided and supported by a TA-RPG facilitator (also referred to in this text as a "therapeutic game master") to collaboratively create compelling stories, overcome challenges, and form bonds as a team. The facilitator will implement specific scenarios within the narrative and/or apply the rules of the game to support participant goals.

TA-RPGs Support Engagement in Treatment and Community

The dual emphasis on flexibility and enjoyment inherent in TA-RPGs due to their play-based nature can support participant engagement in treatment. This enjoyment may increase motivation, engagement, and retention of skills. Indeed, previous studies have found enjoyment to be a significant component of motivation, engagement, and skill retention in child, adolescent, and adult learners (Ares, & Gorrell, 2002, Lucardie, 2014). Further, TA-RPGs are theorized to reduce depression by serving to increase participation in intrinsically rewarding behaviors, as group members become increasingly engaged in a shared and valued activity.

An additional process through which TA-RPGs are thought to produce change is the increased opportunity for interactions, both around the table and within the game. Through their unique pacing, TTRPGs allow for an exaggerated quantity of interactions compared to reality, and provide opportunity for participants to observe the interactions of other people, in a slowed-down, controlled setting. Simply, the more times an individual interacts with novel situations, the more confident and comfortable they become when approaching them.

With regular opportunities for enjoyable, low-stakes social interactions, TA-RPG groups are designed to increase social functioning and engagement in a manner that is consistent with the client's goals and values. TA-RPGs can help individuals to develop and strengthen social networks, as well as appropriately engage other treatment providers and their broader communities.

To illustrate the long-term benefits of TA-RPGs, consider this example of a TA-RPG counseling group within the Psychosocial Rehabilitation and Recovery Center (PRRC) at a VA medical center. Prior to participation, many of the veterans were significantly isolated from others and disengaged from personally valued activities, resulting in regularly missed VA appointments or limited community involvement. One veteran, in particular, presented as considerably anxious, isolated, and paranoid, compared to their descriptions of how they "used to be." Through consistent engagement in the group (i.e., working toward personal goals and sharing their successes alongside their peers), they found their voice again, became more confident, and became more fully engaged in their interpersonal interactions in and outside of the group. Following several months of weekly sessions, the group transitioned from a psychotherapy group into a recreational group. The group determined they would be self-directed, continuing to adventure without the intervention of a therapist, and many of the original members continued to attend the social group within the community instead of at the medical center. As one of the goals of the PRRC is community integration, the group was considered an unqualified success.

Similar to the aforementioned story, TA-RPG groups are particularly appropriate for socially isolated individuals who struggle to engage in typical mental health treatments due to lack of interest, burnout, or social fears. Successful engagement in a TA-RPG group has the capacity to restore hope in successful treatment outcomes, which may improve a participant's willingness to engage in subsequent and auxiliary treatment. Anecdotally, many providers report that their clients become more willing to engage in treatment and demonstrate improved self-advocacy following participation in a TA-RPG group.

Consider the example of John,[1] a "treatment resistant" client and a veteran living in and receiving treatment through a VA domiciliary program. He was noted to be argumentative with other veterans and treatment staff, as well as generally dismissive of treatment and domiciliary rules. John regularly stated he "hated" all therapy groups and thought they were a waste of time. He was referred to a TA-RPG counseling group by his treatment team, with the hopes that a different style of psychotherapy group might better meet his treatment needs and moderate his disruptive behavior. When John initially presented to the group, he was quick to state that he believed he was referred to the group because his case manager "hated" him. He was largely silent during the first session, but began actively participating during the second session (i.e., reading his character sheet, providing recommendations to others regarding their actions, and asking follow-up questions to other clients). During the fourth session, John stated that although he initially thought the group was "stupid," he now viewed it as a viable treatment option, and remarked "I actually find myself looking forward to this group." As John steadily increased his active participation in both the game-play and post-game processing components, he became a valuable sounding board for other participants and began to adjust his feedback toward others to be more kind. John attributed his increased trust and respect for his fellow group members to his opportunities to extrapolate how they might respond to real-world situations by their responses to in-game stimuli. Furthermore, his treatment team provided the feedback that he appeared more engaged and respectful in the settings in which they worked with him (i.e., outside of his TA-RPG group). By seventh session, John began referring other Veterans to the group, stating he believed the group would be beneficial to them as well.

Especially for treatment-fatigued youth who may be resistant to talking to yet another adult or another strange group of peers about their feelings and problems, TA-RPGs allow clients to actively participate in the group while moderating their level of emotional disclosure or engagement. One example of this is Sam, an adolescent who participated in a TA-RPG counseling group. Sam initially presented to the group with the assumption that this would be "just another therapy group." They were immediately caught off guard by the format of the group, as well as the lack of an expectation to share their feelings or "secrets" with the group. Sam initially began playing a character that had a hard time listening to others, and would often run off in direct conflict to the pleas of their fellow group members. As the group progressed, Sam began to share more about their personal life, expressing relief and appreciation for the opportunity to open up at their own pace. Though such experiences can be created within other therapeutic modalities, the dual processes of game and group support clients in shifting their focus from game to group, allowing continued engagement in the therapy without becoming overwhelmed or disengaged.

TA-RPGs Support Skill Building

Though participants may not be haggling with 11 merchants, negotiating with city guards, or casting spells to capture a dragon in their real life, their acquired communication, flexibility, and problem-solving skills are directly applicable in real life. Similar to giving a speech as part of a communications class, the topic of the speech may not be transferable, but the acquired skills and experience are. The consequences of player choices and the skills they develop during play, which rely heavily on visualization and verbalization, linger with the participant and translate into their personal lives.

TA-RPGs are posited to increase cognitive flexibility and support social skill development by providing vicarious scenarios that prompt participants to develop and practice specific skills (e.g., problem-solving skills, frustration tolerance, effective communication skills, and perspective taking). In response to a participant's goal to gain insight into their impulsivity, the GM might design doors that, when opened carelessly (i.e., without checking for traps), explode and injure the character or the entire group of characters. Alternatively, to support a participant who has trouble making simple decisions quickly, the facilitator may provide reinforcement of quick responses over "correct" responses, supporting the participant in their journey to enhance their self-confidence. A participant with the goal to improve their nonverbal communication skills may find their character affected by a spell that temporarily suppresses their voice, requiring them to rely on nonverbal communication for a period of the game. In real-life scenarios, participants may need to rely on multiple skills at once. Similar to real life, scenarios can be designed to support the development of multiple skills in the same encounter. For example, consider a participant who struggles with a low frustration tolerance. A scenario may be designed so that the group or individual participants must try multiple solutions before "solving" the puzzle. The number of attempted solutions required to solve the puzzle could gradually rise with each iteration, providing opportunities to practice regulatory coping skills (e.g., deep breathing), planning (e.g., brainstorming), and playfulness in one's approach to problem solving. In any scenario, the facilitator's intervention may be implicit or explicit, depending on the participants' goals, interest, and developmental capacity. As described in these examples, participants' ability to engage experientially with the game's narrative supports skill acquisition through active learning. Active learning allows participants to directly engage and experiment with new material, and is in direct contrast to the typical school learning format of unidirectional learning, where students receive but do not necessarily engage with new information (Joyner & Young, 2006).

Consider the following story of Jo, a participant with a significant history of rejection and bullying from their peers. Initially, Jo was reluctant to trust others and had developed a pattern of protecting themselves by rejecting others before they could be rejected by their peers. During the TA-RPG group, Jo demonstrated this pattern through the actions of their character—acting aggressively toward other player characters and non-player characters (NPCs), dismissing other client's ideas, and making statements such as "My character only works alone." Feedback from other clients, through their character to Jo's character, was a powerful motivator for affirmation and change. Additionally, the frustration caused by Jo's behavior was consistently mediated by the facilitator via clarifying and probing questions, resulting in increased insight and communication skills for Jo, as well as increased understanding and support from other group members. Over time, Jo began to accept that they would not be rejected by the group, while simultaneously gaining awareness of the frustration caused by their character's actions. Ultimately, Jo learned to collaborate with the team and framed the behavior change as growth for themselves and their character.

TA-RPG Treatment Settings

The diversity of settings to which TA-RPGs have been applied successfully speaks to the adaptability and appropriateness of this intervention across settings and populations. The Game to Grow Method of TA-RPGs began through the delivery of social flourishing groups (referred to then as "social skills groups") designed for youth and emerging adults. These non-clinical groups are best suited for individuals who have challenges connecting with others, forming relationships, building self-esteem, and flexibility. For more details on social flourishing, see Chapter 8. The authors have also used TA-RPG groups in various other settings, including clinical settings, targeting their intervention to the presenting needs of the clients in each setting. As with any intervention, some tailoring must be done to fit the intervention appropriately to each population; however, the core tenets of the intervention remain the same across settings. Individuals trained in the Game to Grow Method have successfully run groups in schools, inpatient and residential treatment settings, private practice, community mental health, and other settings.

Community Settings

The authors implement social flourishing groups in community settings, such as schools, universities, libraries, senior centers, foster agencies, and other accessible locations embedded in close proximity to the specific populations served. These groups provide non-clinical relational support in non-stigmatizing settings.

Community Mental Health

The authors developed programs within a children's advocacy center with children and adolescents who had a history of trauma. These groups were run as adjunctive to individual treatment and helped support social connection and self-esteem as part of their trauma recovery process. Individual therapists of group members reported the group participation often supported participants' willingness to talk in individual therapy.

Medical Centers

The authors developed programs in multiple settings within the Veterans Health Administration including residential PTSD treatment, outpatient treatment for severe mental illness, outpatient treatment for substance use, and mental health integrated within a primary care setting. The format and style of each group was successfully altered in each setting to fit the needs of the population. From these groups emerged several peer-led "alumni groups" that consisted of participants who graduated from the TA-RPG group and wanted to continue engaging in TA-RPGs with their community.

Outpatient Private Practice

The authors have successfully run TA-RPG counseling groups for adolescents in private practice settings. The primary diagnoses in these groups were anxiety and depression related. These groups were well received by participants, who cited an appreciation to explore emotions, communication, and personal challenges through the lens of their character, with opportunities for in-depth processing.

Hospital Groups

The authors have implemented TA-RPGs in hospital settings, bringing relational social play to patients in long-term medical care. Because of health concerns, many patients are unable to receive visitors or engage in social contact with others, so the introduction of TA-RPG (using video conferencing) provided not only a rare and valuable opportunity to play with others but also a context in which to meaningfully connect on shared experiences.

How to Use This Book

The text is intended to both provide a comprehensive understanding of the underlying theories that support the implementation of TA-RPG and offer techniques the reader can use to implement their own TA-RPG practice. Chapters are structured so that the reader will begin by learning what TTRPGs are and how many of the common aspects in TTRPGs can be utilized with therapeutic intent. The next several chapters cover the general theoretical foundations of TA-RPGs and the Game to Grow

Method. Building on this foundation, the following section covers population considerations as well as techniques for case conceptualization, treatment planning, and session design. The final chapters are intended to support the reader to begin their own practice, providing guidelines for recruiting participants and advocating to stakeholders. The Game to Grow Method is complex, and chapters will regularly reference content in other parts of the book. While the chapters are structured intentionally, readers can read chapters out of order, skip around to support their understanding of the material, and forge the path best suited to their unique journey into TA-RPGs.

Note

1 Names and some demographic information of all players and characters mentioned have been changed to protect participant privacy.

References

Abbott, M. S., Stauss, K. A., & Burnett, A. F. (2021). Table-top role-playing games as a therapeutic intervention with adults to increase social connectedness. *Social Work with Groups, 45*(1), 16–31. https://doi.org/10.1080/01609513.2021.1932014

Arenas, D. L., Viduani, A., & Araujo, R. B. (2022). Therapeutic use of role-playing game (RPG) in mental health: A scoping review. *Simulation & Gaming, 53*(3). https://doi.org/10.1177/10468781211073720

Ares, N., & Gorrell, J. (2002). Middle school students' understanding of meaningful learning and engaging classroom activities. *Journal of Research in Childhood Education, 16*(2), 263–277. https://doi.org/10.1080/02568540209594989

Battles, A., Davis, A., Kilmer, J., & Kilmer, E.D. (2021, August 13). Dungeons & Dog tags: Enhancing Veteran Mental Health with TTRPGs [Conference session]. *Therapeutic and Applied Geek and Gaming Summit,* https://taggsummit.org/ as the overall link to the conference.

Berkenstock, J. (2021). *Wizards, warriors and wellness: The therapeutic application of board games.* The Bodhana Group.

Blackmon, W. D. (1994). Dungeons and dragons: The use of a fantasy game in the psychotherapeutic treatment of a young adult. *American Journal of Psychotherapy, 48*(4), 624–632. https://doi.org/10.1176/appi.psychotherapy.1994.48.4.624

Blackmore, C., Tantam, D., Parry, G., & Chambers, E. (2012). Report on a systematic review of the efficacy and clinical effectiveness of group analysis and analytic/dynamic group psychotherapy. *Group Analysis, 45*(1), 46–69. https://doi.org/10.1177/0533316411424356

Boccamazzo, R., & Connell, M. (2019, January). *Dungeons, dragons, and psychology.* Clinician Workshop Presented at Antioch University, Seattle Campus, Seattle, WA.

Bottema-Beutel, K., Park, H., & Kim, S. Y. (2018). Commentary on social skills training curricula for individuals with ASD: Social interaction, authenticity, and stigma. *Journal of Autism and Developmental Disorders, 48*(3), 953–964. https://doi.org/10.1007/s10803-017-3400-1

Burlingame, G. M., Fuhriman, A., & Mosier, J. (2003). The differential effectiveness of group psychotherapy: A meta-analytic perspective. *Group Dynamics: Theory, Research, and Practice, 7*(1), 3–12. https://doi.org/10.1037/1089-2699.7.1.3

Cacioppo, J. T., & Cacioppo, S. (2014). Social relationships and health: The toxic effects of perceived social isolation. *Social and Personality Psychology Compass, 8*(2), 58–72. https://doi.org/10.1111/spc3.12087

Chou, K. L., Liang, K., & Sareen, J. (2011). The association between social isolation and DSM-IV mood, anxiety, and substance use disorders: Wave 2 of the National Epidemiologic Survey on Alcohol and Related Conditions. *The Journal of Clinical Psychiatry, 72*(11), 1515. doi:10.4088/JCP.10m06019gry

Chung, T. (2012). Table-top role playing game and creativity. *Thinking Skills and Creativity, 8*, 56–71. https://doi.org/10.1016/j.tsc.2012.06.002

Connell, M., Kilmer, E. D., & Kilmer, J. N. (2020). Tabletop role playing games in therapy. In A. M. Bean, E. S. Daniel, & S. A. Hays (Eds.), *Integrating geek culture into therapeutic practice: The clinician's guide to geek therapy* (pp. 75–93). Leyline.

Cook, C. R., Gresham, F. M., Kern, L., Barreras, R. B., Thornton, S., & Crews, S. D. (2008). Social skills training for secondary students with emotional and/or behavioral disorders: A review and analysis of the meta-analytic literature. *Journal of Emotional and Behavioral Disorders, 16*(3), 131–144. https://doi.org/10.1177/1063426608314541

Cuijpers, P., van Straten, A., Andersson, G., & van Oppen, P. (2008). Psychotherapy for depression in adults: A meta-analysis of comparative outcome studies. *Journal of Consulting and Clinical Psychology, 76*(6), 909–922. https://doi.org/10.1037/a0013075

Daniau, S. (2016). The transformative potential of role-playing games: From play skills to human skills. *Simulation and Gaming, 47*(4), 423–444. http://doi.org/10.1177/1046878116650765

Dyson, S. B., Chang, Y. L., Chen, H. C., Hsiung, H. Y., Tseng, C. C., & Chang, J. H. (2016). The effect of tabletop role-playing games on the creative potential and emotional creativity of Taiwanese college students. *Thinking Skills and Creativity, 19*, 88–96. https://doi.org/10.1016/j.tsc.2015.10.004

Elms, A. C. (1966). Influence of fantasy ability on attitude change through role playing. *Journal of Personality and Social Psychology, 4*(1), 36–43. https://doi.org/10.1037/h0023509

Eussen, M. L., Van Gool, A. R., Verheij, F., De Nijs, P. F., Verhulst, F. C., & Greaves-Lord, K. (2013). The association of quality of social relations, symptom severity and intelligence with anxiety in children with autism spectrum disorders. *Autism, 17*(6), 723–735. https://doi.org/10.1177/1362361312453882

Frueh, B. C., Turner, S. M., Beidel, D. C., & Cahill, S. P. (2001). Assessment of social functioning in combat veterans with PTSD. *Aggression and Violent Behavior, 6*(1), 79–90. https://doi.org/10.1016/S1359-1789(99)00012-9

Gates, J. A., Kang, E., & Lerner, M. D. (2017). Efficacy of group social skills interventions for youth with autism spectrum disorder: A systematic review and meta-analysis. *Clinical Psychology Review, 52*, 164–181. https://doi.org/10.1016/j.cpr.2017.01.006

Gifford-Smith, M. E., & Brownell, C. A. (2003). Childhood peer relationships: Social acceptance, friendships, and peer networks. *Journal of School Psychology, 41*(4), 235–284. https://doi.org/10.1016/S0022-4405(03)00048-7

Henrich, S., & Worthington, R. (2021). Let your clients fight dragons: A Rapid Evidence Assessment regarding the therapeutic utility of 'Dungeons & Dragons'. *Journal of Creativity in Mental Health*, 1–19. https://doi.org/10.1080/154 01383.2021.1987367

Jones, D. E., Greenberg, M., & Crowley, M. (2015). Early social-emotional functioning and public health: The relationship between kindergarten social competence and future wellness. *American Journal of Public Health*, *105*(11), 2283–2290. https://doi.org/10.2105/AJPH.2015.302630

Joyner, B., & Young, L. (2006). Teaching medical students using role play: Twelve tips for successful role plays. *Medical Teacher*, *28*(3), 225–229.

Kasari, C., Rotheram-Fuller, E., Locke, J., & Gulsrud, A. (2012). Making the connection: Randomized controlled trial of social skills at school for children with autism spectrum disorders. *Journal of Child Psychology and Psychiatry*, *53*(4), 431–439.

Kato, K. (2019). Employing tabletop role-playing games (TRPGs) in social communication support measures for children and youth with autism spectrum disorder (ASD) in Japan: A hands-on report on the use of leisure activities. *Japanese Journal of Analog Role-Playing Game Studies*, 23–28. https://doi. org/10.14989/jarps_0_23

Kilmer, E. D. (2020, July). *Role-playing game therapy in a veteran population* [Presentation]. American Lake VA Medical Center Training Day, Tacoma, WA.

Kilmer, J., & Kilmer, E. D. (2018, July). *Therapeutic benefits of role-playing games* [Address]. Waco VA Community Mental Health Summit, Waco, TX.

Kipper, D. A., & Ritchie, T. D. (2003). The effectiveness of psychodramatic techniques: A meta-analysis. *Group Dynamics: Theory, Research, and Practice*, *7*(1), 13. https://doi.org/10.1037/1089-2699.7.1.13

Low, W. R., Sandercock, G. R. H., Freeman, P., Winter, M. E., Butt, J., & Maynard, I. (2020). Pressure training for performance domains: A meta-analysis. *Sport, Exercise, and Performance Psychology*, *10*(1), 149–163. https://doi.org/10.1037/ spy0000202

Lucardie, D. (2014). The impact of fun and enjoyment on adult's learning. *Procedia - Social and Behavioral Sciences*, *142*, 439–446. https://doi.org/10.1016/j. sbspro.2014.07.696

Mikami, A. Y., Smit, S., & Khalis, A. (2017). Social skills training and ADHD—What works? *Current Psychiatry Reports*, *19*(12), 1–9. https://doi.org/10.1007/ s11920-017-0850-2

Mueser, K. T., & Bellack, A. S. (2009). Social skills training: Alive and well?. *Journal of Mental Health*, *16*(5), 549–552. https://doi.org/10.1080/09638230701494951

Okuda, Y., Bond, W., Bonfante, G., McLaughlin, S., Spillane, L., Wang, E., . . . & Gordon, J. A. (2008). National growth in simulation training within emergency medicine residency programs, 2003–2008. *Academic Emergency Medicine*, *15*(11), 1113–1116. https://doi.org/10.1111/j.1553-2712.2008.00195.x

Orsmond, G. I., Shattuck, P. T., Cooper, B. P., Sterzing, P. R., & Anderson, K. A. (2013). Social participation among young adults with an autism spectrum disorder. *Journal of Autism and Developmental Disorders*, *43*(11), 2710–2719. https://doi.org/10.1007/s10803-013-1833-8

Philipsen, A., Richter, H., Peters, J., Alm, B., Sobanski, E., Colla, M., . . . & Hesslinger, B. (2007). Structured group psychotherapy in adults with attention deficit hyperactivity disorder: Results of an open multicentre study. *The Journal of Nervous and Mental Disease, 195*(12), 1013–1019. https://doi.org/10.1097/NMD.0b013e31815c088b

Rajendran, K., & Videka, L. (2006). Relational and academic components of resilience in maltreated adolescents. *Annals of the New York Academy of Sciences, 1094*(1), 345–349. https://doi.org/10.1196/annals.1376.047

Rosselet, J. G., & Stauffer, S. D. (2013). Using group role-playing games with gifted children and adolescents: A psychosocial intervention model. *International Journal of Play Therapy, 22*(4), 173–192. https://doi.org/10.1037/a0034557

Roy, J. (2019, July 16). VA North Texas group therapy uses storytelling . . . and dragons. *VAntage Point.* Retrieved November 2, 2021, from https://blogs.va.gov/VAntage/62951/va-north-texas-group-therapy-uses-storytelling-and-dragons/

Segrin, C., & Flora, J. (2000). Poor social skills are a vulnerability factor in the development of psychosocial problems. *Human Communication Research, 26*(3), 489–514. https://doi.org/10.1111/j.1468-2958.2000.tb00766.x

Simkins, D. W., & Steinkuehler, C. (2008). Critical ethical reasoning and role-play. *Games and Culture, 3*(3–4), 333–355. https://doi.org/10.1177%2F1555412008317313

Tew, J., Ramon, S., Slade, M., Bird, V., Melton, J., & Le Boutillier, C. (2012). Social factors and recovery from mental health difficulties: A review of the evidence. *The British Journal of Social Work, 42*(3), 443–460. https://doi.org/10.1093/bjsw/bcr076

Tillitski, C. J. (1990). A meta-analysis of estimated effect sizes for group versus individual versus control treatments. *International Journal of Group Psychotherapy, 40*(2), 215–224. https://doi.org/10.1080/00207284.1990.11490601

Tsai, J., El-Gabalawy, R., Sledge, W. H., Southwick, S. M., & Pietrzak, R. H. (2015). Post-traumatic growth among veterans in the USA: Results from the National Health and Resilience in Veterans Study. *Psychological Medicine, 45*(1), 165–179. https://doi.org/10.1017/S0033291714001202

Umberson, D., & Karas Montez, J. (2010). Social relationships and health: A flashpoint for health policy. *Journal of Health and Social Behavior, 51*(1_suppl), S54–S66. https://doi.org/10.1177/0022146510383501

Warren, J. I., Stein, J. A., & Grella, C. E. (2007). Role of social support and self-efficacy in treatment outcomes among clients with co-occurring disorders. *Drug and Alcohol Dependence, 89*(2–3), 267–274. https://doi.org/10.1016/j.drugalcdep.2007.01.009

Wergeland, G. J. H., Fjermestad, K. W., Marin, C. E., Haugland, B. S. M., Bjaastad, J. F., Oeding, K., . . . & Heiervang, E. R. (2014). An effectiveness study of individual vs. group cognitive behavioral therapy for anxiety disorders in youth. *Behaviour Research and Therapy, 57*, 1–12. https://doi.org/10.1016/j.brat.2014.03.007

Wright, J. C., Weissglass, D. E., & Casey, V. (2017). Imaginative role-playing as a medium for moral development. *Journal of Humanistic Psychology*, 1–31. https://doi.org/10.1177%2F0022167816686263

Yalom, I., & Leszcz, M. (2020). *Theory and practice of group psychotherapy* (6th ed.). Basic Books.

2

An Introduction to Tabletop Role-Playing Games

Tabletop role-playing games (TTRPGs) provide a unique type of game experience that differs from many other types of game. This chapter defines and clarifies terms and colloquialisms often found in and around the hobby of TTRPGs as well as the ways these terms are used throughout the book. Additionally, this chapter introduces the in-game roles of participants and facilitators, and outlines the structure of play. TA-RPG facilitators must be familiar with the participation structures of TTRPGs in order to communicate and facilitate the intervention effectively, and should be familiar with many, if not all, of these terms to support cultural fluency with players who may already be steeped in the hobby.

What Is a Tabletop Role-Playing Game?

In TTRPGs, a group of players collaboratively constructs a story together through a mix of pre-determined content, spontaneous role-play, and structured rules. In most TTRPGs, one player takes on a facilitator role (often called a "game master") and guides the other players, who are each playing a character, through a story that responds to the characters' actions. Structured rules dictate the actions that players can take and the outcomes that result. Additionally, many TTRPGS include randomizing agents, such as dice, that help provide a sense of unpredictability and variability to the collaborative experience, determining a range of success and failure to character actions.

TTRPGs vary immensely in structure, style, and presentation. Usually there is one game master (GM), and between two and five players in a game, though some games do not have a GM role. These "GM-less RPGs" are discussed further in Chapter 6. Many games have predetermined genres and story settings that guide the narrative. Some TTRPGs mimic board games or card games, or even video games, in their presentation. For the sake of this text, TTRPG refers specifically to analog (i.e., not electronic) games focused on group collaborative storytelling. Many

DOI: 10.4324/9781003281962-2

analog TTRPGs can be played over a digital medium, such as over video chat, but the basic participation structures remain the same and can be leveraged for TA-RPGs.

The Role of the Player

Each player has a character (often called a "player character") whose mechanics and story can be pre-designed or created by the player. Players typically control only their own individual character, whose choices and actions are the sole decision of that player throughout the course of play. As a story progresses, characters will often grow over time. In addition to the personal growth that might be based in the narrative (e.g., the character becomes more trusting), TTRPGs often contain rules determining how characters acquire new skills, abilities, and benefits as they gain experience (e.g., the character learns how to pick locks).

The Role of the Game Master

The "game master" (often called the "GM") is responsible for introducing the story, describing the environment, adjudicating rules interpretations, and maintaining the timing and engagement of the game. Typically, the game master does not have their own character who participates in the story in the same capacity as the player characters, though the GM portrays any non-player characters (referred to as "NPCs") in the story. To effectively navigate the GM role, the facilitator should have an understanding of the game mechanics, the setting, the story, and each participant's character.

Cycle of Play

TTRPGs typically feature a semi-structured back-and-forth dialogue between the players and the GM. Unlike video games or board games that have a limited number of ways for players to engage, TTRPGs allow players greater opportunities for creativity. Their choices are limited only by the players' imaginations, the outcomes of potential dice rolls, and the rules of the game, which can be adapted flexibly by the GM. Figure 2.1 outlines the actions GMs and players take during a TTRPG encounter.

Describe the Situation (Game Master Action)

The GM sets up the scene, similar to a narrator voice-over at the beginning of a movie. The GM describes pertinent information in the environment, providing both crucial details necessary for the players to

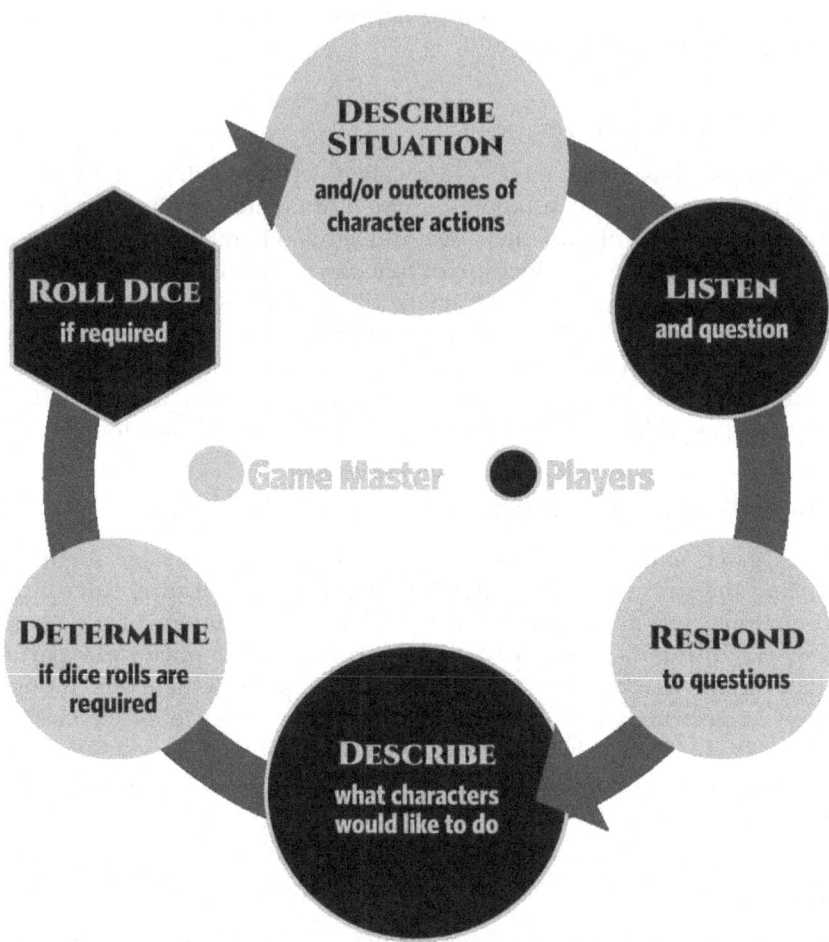

Figure 2.1 Cycle of Play

make decisions and thought-provoking details designed to prompt the imagination of the players. The GM may remind players of their goal and will usually describe obstacles in the characters' way.

> You walk toward the old home in the woods that was marked on your map. There is a large fence around a back portion of the property. The front door is open, slightly, and you step inside. There is old worn furniture strewn about, along with a small stove in the corner. The home is small, consisting only of a single room. There is very little here that looks like it has any value at all. However, your eyes

fall upon an ornate chest in the corner of the room with a distinctive symbol on it. It sticks out like a sore thumb.

Listen and Ask Questions (Player Action)

Players reflect on the GM's description, and have a chance to ask follow-up questions.

> You mentioned the ornate chest has a distinctive symbol on it. Has my character seen this symbol before?
>
> or
>
> You said there is a fence around the back of the property. How tall is it?

Respond to Questions (Game Master Action)

The GM responds and clarifies as appropriate to player questions. The GM may also request dice rolls from the players, if the question that was asked might require specialized knowledge, or ask questions about the player's character to help determine how to answer.

> Your character has seen symbols like this before. You learned in magic school that it is a powerful rune of protection.
>
> or
>
> The fence looks to be about equal to your character's height.

Describe What Characters Would Like to Do (Player Action)

The player describes what action their character would like to do in response. They may reference specific skills, abilities, or weapons on their character sheet, or give a more narrative description.

> I want to try and remember if I know anything more about that symbol.
>
> or
>
> My character tries to open the chest.
>
> or
>
> I run up to the fence, grab the top with my hands, and try to jump over it!

Determine if Dice Rolls Are Required (Game Master Action)

In a TTRPG, the action that was described by the player does not occur in the story until the GM declares it so. The GM may ask clarifying questions and will let the player know if dice rolls are required based on the actions the character is attempting.

In addition to or in lieu of dice rolls, the facilitator may ask the participant to describe or act out the action, prompting further description or story input from the player.

> Do you reach down and open the chest carefully, or attempt to just kick it open? Either way, roll a strength check to see how successful you are.
>
> or
>
> You are such an athletic character that you don't need to roll a check to jump over the fence, but describe a little more what your character looks like as they leap effortlessly over it.

Roll Dice (Player/Game Master Action)

If necessary, the player will roll dice to determine the extent of success or failure of the attempted action. In some scenarios, the facilitator may also roll dice if the environment or an NPC may do something to impede the actions of the character. Most TTRPGs use dice as the randomizing agent of the game. If another tool is used, that would likely take place during this step instead of the dice roll. Diceless games are discussed further in Chapter 6. Depending on the specific game being played, the player may add numbers (often called "bonuses") to their result on the basis of the character's unique abilities.

> I rolled a 5. My character has a bonus of +3, so it is a total of 8 on my check to open the chest.

Describe the Situation (Game Master Action)

Informed by the result of any rolled dice, the GM will determine and describe the outcome of the character's action. If the action has a chance of failure (i.e., the dice roll result is lower than the threshold for success chosen by the GM), they will narrate the outcome and prompt the players to suggest a follow-up action. If the GM determines the action to be successful, they will narrate the result and continue the story.

You kick the chest with all of your might, but it doesn't budge. You watch as the symbol on the front suddenly glows red with magic when your kick lands. It looks like this chest is magically sealed.

or

As you effortlessly leap over the fence—just as you described—you land on a soft material. You can see that the entire yard is completely covered with mushrooms of many varieties.

The Story Continues

As the GM provides subsequent plot details and players continue to make decisions, the narrative continues to expand. Depending on the specific game system being utilized, the game may look very different, though the core gameplay cycle will be fairly consistent across a majority of game systems. Players may gather once to tell a short story, or they may gather many subsequent occasions to continue building a long epic tale. GMs can facilitate stories entirely of their own design, or can utilize a pre-written "adventure module" that will provide a multitude of story details in advance.

TTRPG stories are provided in many genres, including medieval fantasy, horror, cyberpunk, and science fiction (Weinberger, 2021). See Chapter 6 for an overview of many common TTRPG settings. Likewise, the types of adventures and story goals can shift based on group interests. Players can explore a new world, search for hidden treasure, start a business, participate in a journey of romantic discovery, complete quests for interdimensional travelers, and more. The possibilities are limited only by the imaginations of the game participants.

While the TTRPG experience itself manifests as a series of encounters as described in the Cycle of Play, those encounters are sequenced in an overarching storyline. Each time participants get together and play a TTRPG is called a game "session," and small self-contained story arcs that can be completed in one or two sessions is typically called a "one-shot." When players meet multiple sessions to play through a larger story, the story is called an "adventure," though longer adventures are sometimes referred to as "campaigns."

It may aid understanding of game terminology to compare TTRPG play to serialized American television programs. In many such shows, long stories are told through a series of episodes tied together over the course of a "season." A single session of TTRPG play is like a single episode of a serialized TV show, and an adventure may be conceptualized as a season. Many shows feature larger storylines of character growth over the course of several seasons, which are analogous to a TTRPG campaign.

Stories are told in episodes of television shows through a series of subsequent scenes, which are each similar to a single encounter within the game. Many episodes of serialized television shows end on a cliffhanger, leaving the viewer eager to continue watching. Because TTRPG play is unscripted, single sessions of TTRPG gameplay may not regularly have their own complete arcs the same way television shows often do, but players, like viewers, are often left eager to continue the story.

Most GMs facilitate games with materials that have been prepared in advance. They will have some understanding of where the story might go and what actions the player characters may take. When adventures are planned entirely in advance, either by the GM or by another creator, they are often called adventure "modules," though GMs generally use modules as a framework on which to build a story, and rely on player input to shape the way the story progresses. For more information on modules, see Chapters 6 and 13. For an example module, see Chapter 15.

Before implementing therapeutically applied role-playing games (TA-RPGs), TA-RPG facilitators should give important consideration to the selection of game system, adventure content, and adventure and session length, as discussed extensively throughout this book.

Reference

Weinberger, T. (2021, July 7). The most-played tabletop RPGs in 2021. *Drama Dice*. Retrieved July 17, 2022, from www.dramadice.com/blog/the-most-played-tabletop-rpgs-in-2021/#:~:text=What's%20the%20most%20popular%20tabletop,fi%2C%20Cyberpunk%20and%20super%20heroes

3

Common Aspects of Tabletop Role-Playing Games That Support Growth

At this time, there are limited tabletop role-playing games (TTRPGs) that have been designed specifically for therapeutic applications, but most TTRPGs have been designed to support creative and collaborative gameplay (as collaboration in the storytelling process is the goal), and can be effectively utilized in therapeutic applications. TTRPG game mechanics are designed to shape the play of the game and define the style of engagement for both the game master (GM) and the players in order to create compelling stories and memorable play sessions for all participants. For example, clearly defined rules can support participant's engagement and creativity in a game because they reduce the ambiguity and uncertainty and create clear paths for creativity and collaboration.

The aspects of TTRPGs outlined here can be utilized to support therapeutic applications. It is important to note that not all TTRGPs may contain these specific system designs, and it is up to the therapeutic GM to select a game that contains the most appropriate tools for therapeutic potential for their group and participants. This is further discussed in Chapter 6.

Common Goals

In TTRPGs, the players (and their characters) are set up to work together toward shared goals. Instead of each player trying to beat others to the finish, players are often on the same team against a shared obstacle or enemy. This sets participants up to collaborate and work together instead of against each other.

The establishment of common goals helps the individual participants to align together against outside obstacles. This can support the resolution of disagreements between group members and encourage players to use pro-social behaviors, as working together is a necessary component of success within the game (and often outside of the game). Unlike many board games and video games, the design of TTRPGs requires that

DOI: 10.4324/9781003281962-3

all players work together. Thus, in-game goals are often impossible to achieve without this teamwork.

Collaborative Storytelling

Though the GM holds much of the responsibility for describing the world and leading the narrative, the players' responses to the world the GM creates have a tangible impact on the world and storyline. Participants have the ability to change the game world, either through their characters' actions or through their own input. In a TTRPG, this creates a strong sense of engagement with the game and story. It is not just a story that is being told to the player, but one in which the players are working together to actively impact the outcomes and, at times, the very foundations of the story itself.

In much the same way that clients bring conversations and topics into therapy that are especially important to the individual at that moment in time, players in TTRPG groups will bring stories and themes that carry personal meaning into the game. Additionally, this collaborative nature provides a continued opportunity for players to impress their core beliefs, schema, and important self-history into the game itself. A skilled therapeutically applied role-playing game (TA-RPG) facilitator can intentionally utilize this process, asking the right questions of participants which help to craft a world and story filled with opportunities for personal insight and growth for each participant.

When used as an intentional therapeutic tool, the collaborative nature of TTRPGs can develop and reinforce participants' sense of personal agency and beliefs of self-efficacy. In turn, this can increase a sense of self-confidence and a willingness to self-advocate in future situations.

Turn-Taking

Turn-taking systems (most commonly found in combat portions of TTRPGs) can create increased communication structure and clarity around the order in which participant and non-player character (NPC) actions will take place. Though turn-taking systems are not appropriate for all groups during all moments of gameplay, they can scaffold peer communication, planning, and regulation when needed. Game systems that incorporate turn-taking also provide opportunities to experience logical sequencing, helping the players to use critical reasoning and strategic planning. When players are turn-taking in a collaborative game, they can recognize and advocate for each of their individual contributions.

In TA-RPG groups, turn-taking can be leveraged to slow some players down, encouraging them to plan ahead and manage their resources. For players who struggle to speak up during unstructured, open-ended role-play, the clear opportunity to take a turn may support their active participation. They can know in advance that they will be prompted to speak, and will have designated time to prepare a response.

Feedback and Consequences

The cycle of play in TTRPGs creates consistent opportunities for participants to receive immediate feedback through the results and consequences of their character's actions. After players decide on their character's action, the GM determines whether the action succeeds or fails, narrating how the consequences of that outcome play out within the game. In-game consequences provide a valuable opportunity for active learning.

In TA-RPGs, the facilitator's control over the in-game consequences can be a useful tool in supporting the development of participant's cause-and-effect thinking. The facilitator can determine the success criteria of a particular action and adjust the results in accordance to a player's therapeutic goals. The tailored feedback provided by a TA-RPG facilitator allows the player to receive targeted support. Facilitators can also create opportunities for active reflection when actions do not lead to the consequences intended by a player, supporting them to plan more effectively in the future (i.e., "It seems like that didn't get you what you wanted, what approach would you use next time?"). Additionally, after a participant expresses which actions they would like their character to take, the facilitator could pause before the action transpires in the game. The facilitator can use this space to explore likely outcomes with the participant and reflect on alternatives (i.e., "I'm hearing that your character wants to dive into the ocean currently teeming with sharks. What do they expect to happen if they do that?").

Character Creation and Development

Characters are the avatars through which players engage in tabletop role-playing games (TTRPGs). They consist of both mechanical and narrative elements, the specifics of which are determined by the game system. Players can often create custom characters or utilize pre-made characters, depending on the game system. When players create their own characters, they can be tailored to their preferences and goals. Even if the character is pre-generated, players are invited to customize the narrative details (e.g., name, background information, physical characteristics, and personality). This personalization allows players to determine many of the ways their character will interact with the story.

In TA-RPGs, character customization may increase a participant's sense of agency and autonomy in the game. This can help players feel a much greater sense of engagement with their character's successes and failures, as well as with their contributions to the group and narrative arcs of the story. Often, it is this customization of characters, along with collaborative story elements, that make TTRPGs feel more responsive to player's choices and emotionally engaging than video games or board games.

Regarding mechanical character elements, many systems have basic character attributes that help define the strengths and weaknesses of the character, often including qualities such as physical strength, athleticism, physical hardiness, learned knowledge, innate knowledge, and social prowess. Characters can be further defined by their specialized skills or knowledge, such as their knowledge of history or anatomy, skills with lying and deception, or their skill and knowledge of locks. Players are typically afforded an opportunity to assign numerical values to their character's attributes and to their specific skills, creating a set of unique, defining qualities to their character. These numerical values act as modifiers to actions made during the game, increasing or decreasing the character's chance of success. Characters are usually limited in the number of attributes or skills that they can assign, forcing characters to have both strengths and weaknesses. Similar to real life, the focus of expertise in one area can come at the expense of another.

In contrast, narrative character elements are those that help describe the character and their motivations. Narrative elements can include many aspects of a character's background, such as where they grew up, the communities they are affiliated with, their jobs prior to adventuring, and the family and friends who make up their social connections. This can also include information about their core beliefs, character flaws, a guiding mantra, or any other details that may generally describe their personality and values.

Narrative character elements can offer explanation and direction for mechanical character elements. For example, a character who grew up surviving in the woods might have additional bonuses to their knowledge of plants and animals. However, the reverse can be true, where mechanical elements of a character can help inform their narrative design. A player may notice that a character has bonuses to their ability to pick locks, and create a backstory of a life of crime to help explain this set of skills.

Narrative and mechanical elements can work together to create a holistic character whose backstory and mechanics work together to inform the way the character is portrayed. A character may be excellent at deception because they were trained in a royal court full of intrigue (i.e., a narrative explanation of a mechanical element), but they choose to avoid using the skill because it goes against their value of honest communication. Broadly adept at interpersonal communication, the character now seeks to influence others through more prosocial means, such as persuasive argument (i.e., a mechanical explanation of a narrative element). Characters should be complex reflections of humanity, which can be expressed through both narrative and mechanical elements. As players portray those characteristics—including the breadth of character strengths and flaws—they have further opportunities to experience novel perspectives, experiment with their identity, and reflect on these experiences.

Reliance on Others

In most TTRPGs, the players' characters are all part of an "adventuring party" that work together to overcome the challenges in the story. Their backgrounds, strengths, and weaknesses can be different for each character in a group. This variability and diversity of characteristics creates a need for player characters to rely on one another in order to overcome in-game obstacles. In a TTRPG, this variability creates more dynamic, strategic play for the players, encouraging teamwork and cooperation.

In TA-RPGs, this variability creates an opportunity for players to rely on the help of other players. This is especially important for players who frequently try to solve problems on their own, even to the detriment of their personal goals. To help players build awareness of the adventuring party's various strengths, a therapeutic GM can devise specific scenarios in which players must work together through their characters to overcome challenges. This can promote positive interactions between players who might otherwise avoid one another in the play space.

Randomizing Agents

Most TTRPGs rely on a combination of character attributes and random chance, such as dice rolls, to determine the level or success or failure of a player's choice. Randomizing agents add a sense of suspense and unpredictability to TTRPG play. A player's brilliant plan and their character's expertise in the skill do not guarantee success. Randomizing agents force players and GMs alike to react and adjust to the circumstances of each outcome, often creating unexpected and hilarious results.

Randomizing agents play an important role in the discussion of TA-RPGs, as both an outside influence on results and an opportunity for dealing with the frustration of failure. TA-RPG facilitators can use dice rolls as a way of externalizing failure to an outside source. With the roll of the dice, some well-constructed plans may fail, while some poorly constructed ones may succeed. The facilitator can help participants gain awareness of chance and outside influence as a component of planned success or failure. The externalization of failure to the randomizing agent can be particularly helpful for participants who tend to internalize failure, allowing them to attribute the lack of success to a poor dice roll, rather than to a personal flaw. The skilled therapeutic GM can further encourage this kind of externalization, allowing players to continue to take risks and build a stronger sense of safety (i.e., a failure may not be an accurate reflection of personal qualities).

When appropriately utilized, randomizing agents can support a strong sense of resiliency toward the results of failure. TA-RPG facilitators have significant power to shape the story, including the outcomes of failed actions on the parts of the player characters. Therapeutic GMs can focus on demonstrating that a failure may be just as fun or interesting as a success. In this way, both successful and unsuccessful dice rolls can be an exciting continuation of the story, and can help players to build personal resilience to failure within their own lives.

Nuanced Success/Failure Scale

Though in-game outcomes of player choice are sometimes perceived as a binary success/failure, outcomes often have a more nuanced range. Due to the GM's control over the environment and story, and the collaborative nature of the storytelling experience, TTRPGs can interpret both success and failure in a variety of ways. Many systems incorporate rules for extreme failure or extreme success, often informed by the outcomes of dice rolls. However, even this scale has the opportunity for further nuance between the extremes.

Utilizing a broad range of successes and failures helps to support cognitive flexibility and increase participants' ability to see nuance around their own successes and failures. A nuanced scale of success and failure is an important tool to be used by TA-RPG facilitators, who are often in the position to make decisions about the type of feedback a player should receive for their actions.

As an example from a TA-RPG group, consider a player who is struggling to take appropriate risks, often missing opportunities in their lives for advancement and recognition, is playing a character who decides to jump across a ravine, hoping to avoid the spiky rocks at the bottom. For this player, taking such a risk is in line with their treatment goals. If the player rolled low on a dice roll to jump across, the GM may be remiss to allow them to fail outright for fear that the negative consequences would push the player to be even more risk-avoidant. In this circumstance, the GM can leverage the range of success to allow the character to *almost* succeed, clutching to the far edge of the ravine and requiring the assistance of a fellow player. In such a circumstance, the range of outcomes allows the player to be reinforced in their risk-taking without outright abandoning the structure of the game, creating an exciting in-game moment to reinforce the excitement of adventure. More information about implementing a nuanced scale can be found in the "Spectrum of Yes" section in Chapter 11.

Leveling Up

In TTRPGs, characters grow and change over time. In addition to gaining better equipment, they also develop new skills and abilities. In many TTRPGs, this is called "leveling up" and the specific process is dependent on the game system. These processes typically fall into one of two categories: Experience points (XPs), and a form of story or session-based advancement, which is referred to as "milestone" advancement. When using an XP-based leveling system, player characters are granted XP based on specific accomplishments, often through successful encounters (i.e., combat, exploration, and social). Player characters level up when they have earned enough points. Notably, some game systems only define XP values for combat encounters, leaving the GM to determine the XP value for social and exploration encounters, if any is given at all. This may serve to unintentionally reinforce combat-related solutions, especially among players who are more familiar with GMs who rigidly stick to XP systems that reward combat only. With a milestone-based leveling system, players level up when the GM determines characters or players are ready for the next level. This could be after overcoming a significant challenge, due to the growth and knowledge the player characters gained while working through many smaller tasks, or a result of reaching a specific point in a story arc. This method allows the GM to flexibly support and reward participants working together and trying, even if they are not ultimately successful in their original goal.

Some game systems or GMs use session-based milestone advancement, which brings characters to the next level after a predetermined number of sessions, regardless of the content of the session. Though this can support participant attendance, this may be the least engaging and meaningful leveling strategy, as it is not tied to the in-game actions of the participants. Further, it may be particularly problematic in groups where participants have variable control over their attendance (e.g., transportation barriers, medical concerns).

In most TA-RPG groups, facilitators will likely benefit from utilizing group-based leveling up strategies, meaning they keep all group members at the same level, advancing together as a group. Group leveling keeps player characters relatively balanced regarding skills and abilities, as well as support cohesion and a sense of equity in the group. This is especially important in systems where character leveling can drastically increase an individual's power and abilities. When one player character is significantly more powerful than their peers, they have the potential to accomplish many narrative goals by themselves, removing the need to rely on their teammates. Relatedly, one distinctly less powerful player character may struggle to find opportunities for success within the group, feeling like their contributions do not significantly impact outcomes, removing the feeling of the player's agency in the collaborative creation of the story.

4

A Transtheoretical Approach to Therapeutically Applied Role-Playing Games

Effective use of therapeutically applied role-playing games (TA-RPGs) requires the integration of knowledge and training in both psychotherapy and at least one tabletop role-playing game (TTRPG) system. This chapter discusses issues related to competence and ethics TA-RPGs, the transtheoretical approach to treatment in the Game to Grow Method of TA-RPGs, mechanisms for change from several common modalities in psychotherapy, and example applications of each modality within TA-RPGs.

Competence in TA-RPGs

Before running TA-RPG groups, ensuring competence to work with the population being served, as well as proper training in the facilitator's area of expertise, be that psychotherapy or otherwise, is vital. Furthermore, such training should encompass group modalities, as TA-RPGs leverage interpersonal relationships at their core. In addition to providing quality care that does not harm clients, the public perception must be considered. As Dungeons & Dragons (D&D) and other RPGs are used by the general public for entertainment purposes, it is possible that these games may be used inappropriately by laypeople while being labeled as "therapy" or "psychotherapy." Such an occurrence, especially if clients are harmed, risks TA-RPG groups being labeled as dangerous or inappropriate for treatment. This risk could be considered lesser for other treatments that do not have elements commonly used by the public (e.g., prolonged exposure therapy for posttraumatic stress disorder (PTSD)). Though we believe that trained mental health professionals would not dismiss a treatment because of the actions of untrained laypeople, we recognize that the decisions regarding what mental health professionals should or should not do are often in the hands of laypeople, such as organizational administrators or government legislature.

Currently, there is no research to suggest utilizing TA-RPGs in group therapy results in an increased risk of harm compared to traditional

DOI: 10.4324/9781003281962-4

group therapy methods. Two recent reviews of the literature on applied RPGs did not identify areas of risk, but noted the research in this area is still emerging (Henrich & Worthington, 2021; Arenas et al., 2022). Consistent with traditional group therapy methods, clients may experience uncomfortable emotions as a result of engaging in such groups. Clients should not engage in psychotherapeutic TA-RPG groups if they are clinically contraindicated for an individual, and TA-RPG groups should only be run by professionals who are competent in providing such services with the given population.

A notable example of the importance of clinical appropriateness and knowledge of TTRPGs comes from an inpatient unit for male adolescents in the early 1990s. Ascherman, a psychiatrist, described his observations of client's engagement in client-led D&D games with no staff oversight (1993). His observations identify challenges related to the shift in power and relationship dynamics between the clients engaged in D&D and the staff, most of whom had little to no knowledge of D&D. Ascherman also observed that the position of game master (GM) may have exacerbated disruptive behavior of several clients who had schizotypal and narcissistic related diagnoses. In this particular setting, a therapist-facilitated TTRPG group may have supported client/staff relationships as opposed to the ways the client-led group exacerbated relational challenges between clients and staff.

A Transtheoretical Approach

The Game to Grow Method of TA-RPGs is a trans-theoretical approach to psychotherapy that relies heavily on common elements found in many effective psychotherapies. At its core, it is an interpersonal treatment founded on psychological principles involving the intentional intervention of a trained professional in individualized assistance of a client seeking support for a specific issue (Wampold & Imel, 2015). Furthermore, studies examining the effectiveness of numerous psychotherapeutic interventions have found them to be equally effective, especially in reducing general distress and improving quality of life (Luborsky et al., 2002). The Game to Grow Method of TA-RPGs is influenced by both existing psychotherapy interventions and existing game systems. The authors find no need to re-invent very effective wheels, but have worked to meld existing components into a cohesive vehicle for change. This chapter will briefly highlight the mechanism of change from several common schools of thought in psychotherapy.

Although many common theories of change and intervention modalities will be covered in this chapter, an exhaustive list of interventions that can accommodate TA-RPGs is beyond the scope of this work. When utilizing the Game to Grow Method of TA-RPGs within a particular intervention framework, consider the following conceptualization questions:

1. How does the orientation conceptualize problems/challenges?
2. What is the goal of the participant (e.g., increased assertiveness, setting boundaries, increased insight, modify behavior)?
3. How can those goals be supported through the Core Capacities outlined in Chapter 8?
4. What supports does the client need to succeed?
5. How does the facilitator intervene (e.g., Socratic questioning, didactic instruction, experiential learning)?

Acceptance and Commitment Therapy (ACT)

Acceptance and Commitment therapy (ACT, pronounced as the word "act") theorizes that distress and suffering originate from psychological rigidity/inflexibility. This rigidity stems from disconnection from the here and now, unclear values, value-inconsistent behavior, inflexible identity between contexts, treating one's thoughts as reality (fusion), and avoidance (commonly of thoughts and feelings). In response, ACT practitioners work to help clients increase their psychological flexibility through six interrelated factors, known in ACT as the hexaflex. These factors are mindfulness (i.e., being in the moment), identifying personal values, committing action toward those personal values, understanding the self-in-context to one's environment or situation, separating oneself from one's thoughts (defusion), and acceptance of what is (Hayes et al., 2012).

Despite its focus on cognitions and behaviors, ACT differs from traditional cognitive behavioral therapy (CBT) (see later) in its emphasis on noticing and accepting one's thoughts, feelings, sensations, and memories over trying to change or "correct" them. ACT providers work with their clients to identify the "unworkability of excessive and misapplied control to internal experience" (Walser et al., 2012, p. 44). The therapist and client work to counteract control by fostering willingness and openness toward one's internal experiences, which involves acceptance and awareness that one *has* a mind, rather than *is* their mind. ACT therapists further build willingness by helping clients to develop a sense of self that is larger than the content of their thoughts, emotions, and sensations—a sense of an "experiencer," something larger that serves as the context for the many, varied experiences of an individual. ACT posits that once one accepts that they *have* thoughts and feelings, but are *not* their thoughts and feelings, they are free to make values-based choices and take action to move in directions that are consistent with their values.

TA-RPG facilitators who specialize in ACT help their players achieve their therapeutic goals by utilizing the game to foster growth in the six areas of the hexaflex. Participants can be prompted to remain mindful of their bodily sensations, thoughts, and feelings throughout the session, at both the player and character level. Participants are encouraged to remain cognizant of their character's thoughts, feelings, and actions while remaining "defused" from their character. Participants can practice flexibly connecting to and distancing themselves from their character's internal experience, maintaining a healthy aesthetic distance from their character and healthy psychological distance from the content of their thoughts and feelings. Throughout this process, players and characters are encouraged to identify and connect with their values—that is, what they stand for, who they want to be/become, and what they consider most important/precious. Then, they are further encouraged to take actions around the table, in the game, and outside of session that are consistent with their values. A player might apply their own personal values to their character, while another player might create a character with values that are significantly different from their own. Both cases are valid, as they each provide an opportunity to gain exposure to and experience with acting flexibly and consistently with a set of values—using their character to observe what it could look like and feel like to have greater consistency between values and behavior.

Cognitive Behavioral Therapy

CBT is among the most utilized modalities in psychotherapy (Barkham et al., 2021). CBT therapists collaborate with clients to replace maladaptive thoughts and behaviors with more adaptive patterns that are in line with client's personal goals (Beck, 2011). According to cognitive theory, distress and suffering are posited to stem from maladaptive automatic thoughts/beliefs. These thoughts often involve negative beliefs about oneself, other people, the world, and the future. Although maladaptive thoughts may be considered "unrealistic" or "unhelpful," they nevertheless influence undesired emotional and behavioral responses in the experiencer. The cognitive model seeks to synthesize the relationship between situations (events), automatic thoughts/beliefs, and reactions (i.e., emotions, behaviors, physiological responses). More specifically, from the lens of CBT, an event does not inherently elicit a specific response. Instead, it is the perception or interpretation of the event that directly influences one's response. Therefore, identifying, challenging, and rebalancing maladaptive beliefs to be fairer and more accurate become one of the primary vectors for change in CBT. In addition to the emphasis on cognitions, CBT also strives to identify the nature and function (i.e., the reason, purpose, or motivation) of behavior in a person's life. All behaviors are assumed to serve one or multiple functions for an individual, and perhaps most importantly, are contextually derived.

TA-RPG facilitators who specialize in CBT work with participants by providing narrative scenarios designed to identify and challenge maladaptive thoughts, as well as to provide a space to observe, process, and ultimately correct maladaptive behavior. For example, a player may experience a situation wherein their thoroughly devised plan to sneak into a vault falls apart, resulting in the party being caught by guards and thrown in jail. The player may respond by thinking to themselves (and/ or voicing aloud), "I can never do anything right." Such a belief is likely to result in that player feeling sad and angry toward themselves. Indeed, an understandable response if such a thought accurately reflected reality. A cognitive behavioral therapist would work with such a client to identify the evidence for and against such a belief, review facts and context, determine the presence of patterns of problematic thinking (e.g., jumping to conclusions; emotional reasoning), and rewrite the thought to be more balanced and accurate ("There are some things that I do very well, some things that I struggle with, and many things I am still learning to do better"). In a game session, the facilitator may reference prior game sessions that directly contradict the thought "I can never do anything right," resulting in opportunities to explore challenging questions such as "Is that belief a fact, or merely something you commonly say to yourself?" Additionally, future scenarios can be used to contradict, compliment, or complicate one's beliefs about themselves, other people, and the world—ultimately providing corrective experiences that can be leveraged to influence more balanced and adaptive beliefs.

TA-RPGS also provide a context for facilitators and participants to gain insight into maladaptive behaviors before providing a space to rehearse more adaptive replacement behaviors. For example, the party has been speaking with a powerful wizard, from whom they have received a quest and are now engaged in asking clarifying questions as to the nature of the quest. One player becomes bored and, eager to end the current scene and move the narrative forward, starts a fire in the wizard's home. The conversation with the wizard ends and the party moves on, but with frustration toward the player who started the fire. In this scenario, the maladaptive behavior is to cause a significant disruption (i.e., starting a fire), with the function of transitioning into a more interesting scene. Of course, the GM could simply request the player cease the target behavior, but such an intervention is unlikely to be successful if the target behavior is not replaced with a new, adaptive behavior that serves a similar function. Instead, the player could be introduced to assertive communication techniques, which could be prompted and practiced within the game during similar situations (e.g., expressing "I am bored, can we move on," or "what can I do to prepare while y'all are speaking to the wizard?"). TA-RPGs provide a unique environment for the rehearsal of new behaviors, allowing participants to observe potential responses to their actions, without also having to contend with the consequences associated with a higher risk environment (e.g., at work or school).

Dialectical Behavior Therapy

Dialectical Behavior Therapy (DBT) is a skill-focused modality designed to teach clients adaptive ways to manage difficult emotions and develop healthy interpersonal relationships (Linehan, 2014). Although originally developed to treat individuals with borderline personality disorder, DBT has been found effective in treating a broad range of disorders. DBT skills can be categorized into four core domains: mindfulness, distress tolerance, emotional regulation, and interpersonal effectiveness. Mindfulness skills target awareness, acknowledgment, and acceptance of one's internal and external environment and aim to help clients remain focused on the present moment. Distress tolerance skills aim to decrease maladaptive patterns of escape and avoidance by increasing one's ability to endure unpleasant emotions. Emotion regulation skills focus on techniques to identify, describe, manage, and alter problematic emotionality. Finally, interpersonal effectiveness skills cover strategies to enhance communication in respectful and assertive ways.

DBT is influenced by the concept of dialectics in philosophy—the art of examining and balancing opposite perspectives. This modality accommodates the necessity of complexity and nuance by guiding clients to learn to hold conflicting perspectives, challenge binary thinking (i.e., black and white thinking; all-or-nothing thinking), and find balance to promote acceptance and growth (Linehan, 2014). DBT treatment is commonly a combination of individual therapy to address motivation, treatment barriers, and skill application, with group therapy to learn and practice skills within a collaborative, social context. However, administration of DBT can vary, providing opportunities for some clients to exclusively attend individual or group sessions without the other.

TA-RPG facilitators who specialize in DBT may integrate DBT skills training throughout treatment. Due to the interactive nature of TA-RPGs, opportunities to practice interpersonal effectiveness will occur throughout the process. Facilitators are able to use both themselves and non-player characters (NPCs) to model self-respect, as well as prompt participants at appropriate moments to consider ways to act in self-respectful ways. Further, NPCs can variably demonstrate respect toward others as a way to model respectful engagement or elicit assertive communication and boundary setting in the characters they interact with.

Facilitators can prompt participants to engage in mindfulness training for several minutes prior to beginning each play session, increasing player capacity to regulate attention toward the present moment in a nonjudgmental fashion. Further, environmental awareness through the five senses can be developed at both the player level and character level, as the GM works to highlight character sensory awareness through elaborate descriptions of in-game environments. Groups of participants eager to engage in skill checks (i.e., perception and insight) may be incentivized to engage in additional moments of mindfulness around the table to earn additional bonuses to such skill checks.

Facilitators may be mindful of moments of narrative tension, wherein characters are expected to be under significant distress. Participants can be prompted to practice distress tolerance skills by guiding their characters through radical acceptance of difficult situations while dungeoneering, to ascribe meaning and benefit to surviving trials and tribulations, and to practice grounding and soothing techniques for in-game benefits for the ultimate purpose of calmly recognizing and wisely responding to difficult situations. Additionally, emotion regulation skills can be encouraged by identifying and labeling emotions at both the player and character level, as well as identifying obstacles to their character's emotional regulation (e.g., triggers that lead to distress) and working as a group to problem-solve workable solutions. Further, opportunities to create pleasant emotional experiences and plan viable coping mechanisms can be integrated into the group's check-in process at the start of each session.

Drama Therapy

Drama therapy, broadly understood as the systematic and intentional use of drama games, narrative activities, and theatrical performance for insight, growth, and change, includes a wide berth of approaches (Gallo-Lopez & Rubin, 2012). Some practitioners focus on written scenes, rehearsals, and self-revelatory performance; others focus on high-intensity improvised dramatic play and the emergence of salient personal material in the "magic circle" of the narrative playspace. Across drama therapy approaches is an emphasis on narrative metaphor, embodied enactment, and a process of "witnessing" either by the self or a designated other. This experiential modality requires participants to take an active role in their treatment as they devise dramatic scenarios, rehearse and/or improvise scenes, construct alternate outcomes, and process the rich metaphorical content of the narrative. Drama therapists additionally focus on enhancing clients' spontaneity and building their role repertoire to help them respond more adaptively and confidently to their presenting circumstances.

The Game to Grow Method of TA-RPGs, as outlined in Chapter 5, is heavily informed by drama therapy and many of the techniques outlined in this book can be considered a drama-therapeutic approach to

TA-RPGs. Drama therapists engaging in TA-RPGs leverage the narrative elements of RPGs as the primary mediums for growth and change, conceptualizing the game primarily as a collaboratively constructed narrative experience rich with opportunities for playful improvisation, projection, and externalization. When appropriate, facilitators can encourage their participants to embody their character, guiding them to enact the character's physical demeanor and speak as the character using their unique vocal quality. Doing so develops characters as external narrative elements, creating an "I-as-character" role distinct from their role as player and role as participant. The facilitator creates in-game story scenarios analogous to real-world experiences and then uses the liminal quality of the TTRPG playspace to guide players to personal insight by reflecting on their roles as character and player, often recognizing maladaptive or problematic interaction patterns that are analogous to or informed by their own experience, or identifying strengths they did not know they had. The facilitator can also guide the participant to integrate those aspects of the character and player roles that the participant desires into a more cohesive self-concept, building confidence and a sense of self-efficacy.

Gestalt Therapy

Gestalt therapy seeks to alleviate suffering by enhancing self-awareness (i.e., mindfulness) through a focus on the present moment (Perls et al., 1951; Nevis, 2014). It is influenced by a number of psychological theories, including person-centered, cognitive, interpersonal, and multisystemic approaches, as well as art and drama therapy. Gestalt therapy posits that human suffering stems from unresolved emotions and unfinished business—rigidly stuck, segregated and unexpressed, in the past. Indeed, the word "gestalt" means "whole," and gestalt therapy asserts that humans ideally function as a coherent unity of mind, body, and culture. Clients are encouraged to process past events by re-experiencing or re-enacting them in the present, instead of merely talking about them. Such an approach encourages clients to experience the (unresolved) emotions of the past in the present moment in order to fully process, resolve, and integrate them into a coherent and holistic experience. Through this process, clients learn to acknowledge the mind–body connection, identify how their own negative thought patterns and behaviors impact their physical and mental health, accept responsibility for and consequences of their behaviors, and learn to meet their own needs within a broader social context.

Gestalt therapists frequently utilize techniques that incorporate role-play, guided imagery, and dreams with a playfully experimental approach. Providers should be mindful that re-experiencing certain events in a group context can be harmful and inappropriate, as the presentation of some content can trigger unanticipated and undesired emotions. However, with consent, clinician guidance, and adequate coping skills among participants, re-enactments can be immensely helpful by providing opportunities for insight, catharsis, and growth. Before using such techniques, the facilitator should be competent in the use of these techniques within a group setting. Within TA-RPGs, facilitators who specialize in gestalt may integrate players' past and current struggles into the narrative of the game, bringing them to life and allowing players new opportunities to gain insight, resolve conflicts, as well as to engage in their own experimentation of new behaviors. Due to gestalt therapy's emphasis on present experience, a facilitator may ask questions to participants mid-game, such as "What are you feeling at this moment?" and "What is your character perceiving, thinking, and feeling right now?"

TA-RPG facilitators who specialize in gestalt therapy directly encourage players to experiment with novel actions for the purpose of supporting novel experiences, ultimately creating opportunities for increased flexibility in relating to oneself and others. Similar to the empty chair technique, facilitators may prompt participants to collaboratively characterize NPCs to reflect relevant characteristics of important figures in a participant's life (e.g., a school bully, a critical family member), aspects of a participant's personality, or specific emotions for the purpose of re-enacting a "direct" interaction to resolve their feelings. In another context, a participant may struggle with implementing an underdeveloped skill (e.g., setting boundaries). In support of this participant, the facilitator could encourage a participant to practice setting boundaries in-game with other characters, or role-play an NPC giving an exaggerated speech about how "useless" boundaries are to encourage a counter argument from the participant. During role-play, the facilitator pays attention to tone and nonverbal behaviors (e.g., gestures, breathing, posture, expression) in order to direct attention toward how such behavior may shift across contexts and to prompt participants to repeat themselves in an exaggerated manner to gain insight into how nonverbal behavior impacts communication.

Humanistic Therapy

Humanistic therapy, including existential and person-centered approaches, posits that one's suffering originates from a discrepancy between a person's actual self and their ideal self (Schneider et al., 2015). This approach to therapy acknowledges that individuals possess personal needs and motivations, choices of action, and the capacity for self-direction and personal insight.

Central to humanistic theory are several core assumptions. The first assumption is that humans possess free will (aka personal agency) and are responsible for their actions and associated consequences. Although burdensome in nature, taking responsibility for one's actions leads to feelings of empowerment and control, contributing to an increasing sense of one's influence on the world. The second assumption is that people are inherently good and are driven to realize their full potential, overcome adversity, produce, advance, and contribute to the world around them. The third assumption is that each person possesses a unique and valid perspective from which they view the world around them. This individualized perspective results in a subjective perception and interpretation of the world, often influencing one's inner experiences and behaviors more strongly than objective reality.

Humanistic therapists work collaboratively with their clients to build insight, self-awareness, and mindfulness of their worldview to enhance empathy, self-compassion, and self-acceptance. Further, they adopt a non-pathologizing view of the participant and assert that an individual client is the expert regarding their own experience of the world. In keeping with the aforementioned assumptions, humanistic therapists elicit change in their clients through the conveyance of unconditional positive regard, empathy, and genuineness (authenticity) in their presentation.

TA-RPG facilitators who specialize in a humanistic perspective may be inclined to take a less directive approach in the narrative compared to the players, empowering them to be more engaged in the building and direction of the world and story. Freedom of choice is heavily emphasized in session to encourage personal agency and responsibility. In this context, participants of TA-RPGs move toward self-actualization through their choices within the narrative. With unconditional positive regard, facilitators assume participants (and their associated characters) are capable of making healthy decisions for themselves, based on the information available to them at the time of action. Participants are encouraged to adopt a similar assumption, as well as encouraged to foster a healthy and stable sense of self through reflection upon their (and their character's) perspectives, motivations, and values. Finally, facilitators honor the assumption that subjective perception outweighs objective reality. Therefore, they encourage participants to view vicarious experiences, and the lessons derived from them, as powerful vectors for growth congruent with direct experiences outside of the game.

Interpersonal Psychotherapy

Interpersonal Psychotherapy (IPT) was developed to treat mood disorders (e.g., major depressive disorder) through enhancement of social functioning and interpersonal relationships (Weissman et al., 2017). IPT specifically seeks to address difficulties related to social isolation, unresolved grief, adjusting to life transitions, and interpersonal conflict (Cuijpers et al., 2016). Similar to CBT, maladaptive cognitions and behaviors are acknowledged and treated, but only to the extent that they impact interpersonal functioning. Individual and group treatment through this modality typically includes an assessment of symptoms and social history prior to a focus on interpersonal functioning and dynamics. Participation in group therapy optimizes access to a stable environment for practicing pertinent social skills.

Although originally applied to adult populations, IPT has been adapted to be applied to adolescent populations (IPT-AST; Young et al., 2012, 2016). TA-RPG facilitators who specialize in IPT may encourage adolescent participants to collaborate with each other to create shared narrative experiences that address common issues such as leaving home/parents, process death, and conflict resolution. For example, the facilitator could introduce a storyline in which the adventuring party inherits an adventuring company, forcing them to adjust to new roles and responsibilities and take on new positions of leadership. In this scenario, the group members would need to work together to distribute responsibilities, determine priorities for their organization, and handle disputes between employees. Throughout treatment, facilitators may prompt participants to draw connections between interpersonal dynamics and mood, practice assertive communication, and collaborative problem solving.

Psychodynamic Therapy

Psychodynamic therapy is a form of treatment influenced by the theories and principles of psychoanalysis (Shedler, 2010). In addition to focusing on the relationship between client and therapist, psychodynamic therapy also directs considerable attention toward how the client relates to the world around them. Psychodynamic therapy is commonly used to treat individuals with depression and related conditions who struggle to develop healthy relationships and who experience a perceived loss of purpose or meaning in their life. During treatment, clients are typically encouraged to explore any topic that occurs to them, such as struggles, hopes, fears, and dreams. Many interventions within this modality focus on increasing insight and correcting undesired, contradictory, and/or unresolved feelings to improve quality of life and decrease the severity of symptoms. Emphasis is placed on assisting clients in resolving current issues by exploring the connection between patterns within current interpersonal functioning, behavior, and thoughts with unresolved issues from the past.

TA-RPG facilitators who specialize in a psychodynamic approach are able to leverage many of this modality's techniques through the process of character creation and the subsequent play of the character. Clients may be encouraged to use free association when creating a character, alter a contemporary version of themselves to fit into a fantasy setting, create an idealized version of oneself, create the opposite of how they perceive themselves, or be prompted to create a character of a certain archetype (e.g., rogue, hero, jester). In this process, they may be encouraged to reflect upon their character's core personality traits, ideals, bonds, flaws, hopes, fears, and insecurities. Regardless, the process of character creation is inherently projective in nature, with players using personal experiences to inform their decisions at both the conscious and unconscious levels. Facilitators may be mindful of how players relate to their environment (i.e., other players and the GM), as well as how they relate to their character. Further, as both character creation and character behavior are informed by projective processes, facilitators may give significant attention toward how a player's character relates to the world and people around them, finds meaning in their life, and makes decisions. Indeed, analyzing a character as a case study can serve as a model of psychodynamic theory that players can apply at a personal level. This particular analysis may be best performed within individual therapy when the focus is on a player character, and within group therapy when the focus is on an NPC.

Narrative Therapy

Narrative therapy seeks to alleviate suffering by helping individuals to separate themselves from their problems through an emphasis on stories, or narratives (Malinen et al., 2013). As individuals accrue experiences and interact with others, they ascribe meaning to those experiences, which ultimately impacts how an individual perceives their own identity and the world around them. Throughout narrative therapy, clients are encouraged to view themselves as experts on the content of their lives as they work to identify, voice, and explore life events and the meaning they have placed upon them. Through this intervention, clients take on the role of narrator and observer of their stories, allowing them to create psychological distance between themselves and their stories. This process of creating distance is known as externalization and affords individuals new perspectives, empowering them to better understand and alter maladaptive thought patterns and behaviors. Further, this new perspective helps clients to revise the narrative of their life to include a future that accommodates and reflects identity, abilities, and purpose independent of their problems. Finally, narrative therapists aim to help their clients frame problem-focused stories within a broader sociocultural context and to make space for other stories and perspectives.

TA-RPG facilitators who specialize in narrative therapy are likely to challenge their players to mindfully reflect upon and retell in-game narratives from multiple perspectives (e.g., the player, their character, the villain, an NPC). Further, these stories can be compared and contrasted with the perspectives of others in the group to enhance insight and empathy. Players may be asked to look for parallels between in-game narratives and real-life experiences. By focusing on in-game stories and their relationship within the broader sociocultural context of the fantasy world, players are able to practice the skills of narrative therapy by first applying them to their character before applying them to their own experiences.

Solution-Focused Therapy

Solution-focused therapy (SFT), also referred to as solution-focused brief therapy (SFBT), helps clients to achieve desired behavioral change by shifting focus away from problems and toward the identification of prior effective solutions and the construction of new solutions (Iveson, 2002; Kim, 2013; O'Connell, 2016). It is designed to be short-term, pragmatic, hope-friendly, and goal-oriented as clients foster unambiguous, succinct, and sensible goals throughout the entire behavioral change process (i.e., formulation, motivation, achievement, and sustainment of change). This process begins by helping clients to produce a detailed description of how their life would be different in either the absence of the problem or upon a significant improvement of the problem. Next, practitioners work with clients to reflect upon their previous experiences and current skills to identify resources and develop realistic and tenable solutions the client can immediately implement. When reflecting upon previous experiences of the problem, emphasis is placed on examining "exceptions"—moments from the client's past when the problem was successfully resolved or managed.

TA-RPG facilitators who specialize in SFT utilize a number of concepts and tools that can be readily applied to TA-RPGs. Goal development questions are used to elicit a client's best hope for how their life will change as a function of attending therapy. This process often includes a detailed description of what a client's life will look like following the achievement of their goal(s). One example of a goal development question is the Miracle Question, which prompts the client to begin imaging a future where the problem is already solved. This question frequently assumes the problem is miraculously solved overnight, while the client is asleep, and asks the client to imagine waking up the following day, to identify the small signs that would indicate the miracle occurred, and to envision the behavioral changes that would naturally occur as a function of the miracle. Responses to this question serve to inform prudent goals, invite reflection upon past experiences that mimic the miracle description, and encourage replication of such exceptions in daily life. Participants of TA-RPGs can be encouraged to apply their personal answers to the Miracle Question to their character's behavior to prompt deeper exploration of behavioral changes associated with the miracle description. Further, players can be encouraged to imagine asking their character the Miracle Question, gaining exposure to and insight into goal development questions from a distance.

Scaling questions are used to help a client assess their bearing, current progress toward their goal, and next steps. Clients are first prompted to rate variables such as their motivation, confidence, or readiness to act associated with their goals. Next, clients are asked to describe necessary changes that would shift their ratings to be one step closer to their goal. This is often an interactive process throughout treatment and facilitators can work with clients to assess and promote growth and change through scaling questions at both the player and character level.

Coping questions are often presented to clients during SFT as a prompt to inspire creative solutions and as a reminder that clients regularly engage in useful behaviors when coping with their problems. Despite significant hardship, many individuals continue to manage their daily lives and accomplish tasks that require considerable effort in the context of distress and/or impairment. TA-RPG facilitators who specialize in SFT can ask coping questions such as "How have you managed to endure thus far?" or "How have you kept things from becoming worse or unmanageable?" toward the player, their character, and potential NPCs. Further, parallels can be drawn between the answers of the player and their character to build insight, allow for new perspectives, and highlight the player's awareness of their own resiliency and resolve.

Conclusion

Successful implementation of TA-RPGs is derived from the integration of training in both the clinical application of psychotherapy and a nuanced understanding of at least one TTRPG game system. Therapeutic GMs are bound by the code of ethics associated with their mental health license to protect clients from harm, provide quality care, and remain within their competency to maintain trust in the eyes of the public. The Game to Grow Method of TA-RPGs is a transtheoretical approach to treatment, as it leverages common elements found throughout many evidence-based treatments and can be flexibly adapted to accommodate a variety of theoretical orientations. In this chapter, mechanisms of change from common schools of thought in psychotherapy were reviewed. Examples from each modality were applied to TA-RPGs to aid psychotherapists interested in integrating TA-RPGs into their practice.

References

Arenas, D. L., Viduani, A., & Araujo, R. B. (2022). Therapeutic use of role-playing game (RPG) in mental health: A scoping review. *Simulation & Gaming, 53*(1), 285–311. https://doi.org/10.1177/10468781211073720

Ascherman, L. I. (1993). The impact of unstructured games of fantasy and role playing on an inpatient unit for adolescents. *International Journal of Group Psychotherapy, 43*(3), 335–344. https://doi.org/10.1080/00207284.1993.11732597

Barkham, M., Lutz, W., & Castonguay, L. G. (Eds.). (2021). *Bergin and Garfield's handbook of psychotherapy and behavior change* (7th ed.). John Wiley & Sons.

Beck, J. S. (2011). *Cognitive behavior therapy: Basics and beyond* (2nd ed.). The Guilford Press.

Cuijpers, P., Donker, T., Weissman, M. M., Ravitz, P., & Cristea, I. A. (2016). Interpersonal Psychotherapy for mental health problems: A comprehensive meta-analysis. *American Journal of Psychiatry, 173*(7), 680–687.

Gallo-Lopez, L., & Rubin, L. C. (Eds.). (2012). *Play-based interventions for children and adolescents with autism spectrum disorders.* Routledge.

Hayes, S. C., Strosahl, K. D., & Wilson, K. G. (2012). *Acceptance and commitment therapy: The process and practice of mindful change* (2nd ed.). The Guilford Press.

Henrich, S., & Worthington, R. (2021). Let your clients fight dragons: A Rapid Evidence Assessment regarding the therapeutic utility of 'Dungeons & Dragons'. *Journal of Creativity in Mental Health,* 1–19. https://doi.org/10.1080/15401383.2021.1987367

Iveson, C. (2002). Solution-focused brief therapy. *Advances in Psychiatric Treatment, 8*(2), 149–156.

Kim, J. S. (2013). *Solution-focused brief therapy: A multicultural approach.* SAGE.

Linehan, M. M. (2014). *DBT skills training manual* (2nd ed.). The Guilford Press.

Luborsky, L., Rosenthal, R., Diguer, L., Andrusyna, T. P., Berman, J. S., Levitt, J. T., Seligman, D. A., & Krause, E. D. (2002). The Dodo bird verdict is alive and well—mostly. *Clinical Psychology: Science and Practice, 9*(1), 2–12. https://doi/10.1093/clipsy.9.1.2

Malinen, T., Cooper, S. J., & Thomas, F. N. (2013). *Masters of narrative and collaborative therapies: The voices of Andersen, Anderson, and White.* Routledge.

Nevis, E. C. (Ed.). (2014). *Gestalt therapy: Perspectives and applications.* CRC Press.

O'Connell, B. (2016). *Solution-focused therapy.* SAGE.

Perls, F., Hefferline, R., & Goodman, P. (1951). *Gestalt therapy: Excitement and growth in the human personality* (New ed.). The Gestalt Journal Press.

Schneider, K. J., Pierson, J. F., & Bugental, J. F. T. (Eds.). (2015). *The handbook of humanistic psychology: Theory, research, and practice* (2nd ed.). SAGE.

Shedler, J. (2010). The efficacy of psychodynamic psychotherapy. *American Psychologist, 65*(2), 98.

Walser, R. D., Sears, K., Chartier, M., & Karlin, B. E. (2012). *Acceptance and Commitment Therapy for Depression in Veterans: Therapist manual.* U.S. Department of Veterans Affairs.

Wampold, B. E., & Imel, Z. E. (2015). *The great psychotherapy debate: The evidence for what makes psychotherapy work* (2nd ed.). Routledge.

Weissman, M. M., Markowitz, J. C., & Klerman, G. L. (2017). *The guide to Interpersonal Psychotherapy* (Expanded, Updated ed.). Oxford University Press.

Young, J. F., Kranzler, A., Gallop, R., & Mufson, L. (2012). Interpersonal Psychotherapy-Adolescent Skills Training: Effects on school and social functioning. *School Mental Health*, *4*(4), 254–264. https://doi.org/10.1007/s12310-012-9078-9

Young, J., Mufson, L., & Schueler, C. (2016). *Preventing adolescent depression: Interpersonal Psychotherapy-Adolescent Skills Training*. Oxford University Press.

5

Foundations of the Game to Grow Method of Theoretically Applied Role-Playing Games

The Game to Grow Method of Therapeutically Applied Role-Playing Games (TA-RPGs) was developed over a decade of practice, informed by the diverse training and experience of the development team and based on established therapeutic approaches. The Game to Grow Method of TA-RPG is a collaborative and fun experience in which participants are collectively and individually guided and supported to maintain a therapeutically beneficial resonance with the characters, plot, and story elements of a tabletop role-playing game (TTRPG). Participants experience reciprocal successes and failures according to a formal set of rules and guidelines that are applied flexibly on the basis of participant need. To put it simply, the Game to Grow Method of TA-RPG is developmental, relational, scaffolded, aesthetically distanced, play-based narrative transference. These six core foundations of the method are applicable regardless of the therapeutic orientation or theory of change from which facilitators approach TA-RPGs.

Narrative Transference

The concept of transference, based on early psychoanalytic theory, can be understood as the displacement or projection of unconscious or subconscious thoughts, feelings, and desires onto something other than its original target (American Psychological Association [APA], n.d.). Alternatively, it has been defined as when an individual uses past experiences to interpret and respond to current situations (Prasko et al., 2010). Per its original conceptualization, transference was typically understood to occur when a therapy client projected their unprocessed feelings about a significant relationship (e.g., a parent/child relationship) onto the relationship with their therapist. Processing transference in therapy brings thoughts and feelings that may unknowingly be causing distress to the client to their conscious attention, allowing the client opportunities to work through unresolved issues and gain insight about themselves.

DOI: 10.4324/9781003281962-5

Similar to other therapeutic approaches, such transference can occur within approaches that utilize TA-RPGs. However, participants of TA-RPGs are considerably more likely to experience another kind of transference known as *narrative* transference. The concept of narrative transference is defined as "the displacement or projection of one's unconscious thoughts, feelings, and desires onto the characters, plot, and story elements of a narrative." Thus, the participants' relationship history, personal experiences, and lived context will influence the ways in which they relate to the narrative. This may manifest in other forms of narrative media as well, such as when someone reads a book, watches a movie, or enjoys any other form of narrative media and feels an emotional resonance with the narrative content on the basis of their own lived experience (e.g., a family drama may be more emotionally evocative for a viewer if it prompts them to consider their own family). In addition to content, narrative transference can also occur with characters. Similar to a parasocial relationship (Horton & Wohl, 1956), narrative transference with a character occurs when strong feelings of identification or admiration may exist between a media consumer and a character in the media that does not actually exist.

Narrative transference can occur between participants and any of the fictional characters in a TTRPG. Narrative transference may also occur in TTRPGs when a participant connects their own lived experience to the content of the plot (e.g., when obstacles, goals, or other in-game challenges mimic real-life experiences) or the other story elements (e.g., theme, tone, setting, conflict). In TTRPGs, players are active participants, not passive consumers, which increases the frequency of opportunities to connect with narrative elements in real time. Unique to TTRPGs, participants can interact with all of the characters in the make-believe context of the game. Additionally, because players create their own characters and are invited to actively collaborate to build the story they are participating in, they are continually prompted to project their own latent thoughts, feelings, and desires onto the evolving narrative. In time, they create a narrative that uniquely reflects the lived experiences of the individual participants and the group as a whole.

The Game to Grow Method posits that narrative transference within the context of TA-RPGs (e.g., players' choice of character, choice of character actions, and responses to in-game content) is an integral component of therapeutic work. Further, processing moments of narrative transference with participants prompts opportunities for growth and elicits insight into their own desires and needs. This process allows participants to extrapolate the insights and growth they experience in group to their lives outside of the groups.

With a facilitator intentionally guiding the narrative experience, narrative transference can be initiated and adjusted by the game master

(GM) for therapeutic impact. Facilitators can incorporate narrative content in order to prompt narrative transference (e.g., an in-game scenario involving a conversation with a belittling authority figure that resembles a participant's employer). As the player interacts with the simulacra, they will experience transference that can prompt insight, growth, and change. The guidance from a facilitator is essential to the Game to Grow Method, and many of the tools in this text are designed specifically with this in mind.

A Tale From the Real-World Table

The therapeutic GM was guiding the players through a fantasy story that involved a global calamity. Plants all over the world were becoming sentient and were taking over. The plants were vying to return the globe to an "age of green," a time from long before when plants reigned supreme. In order to defeat the plants, the protagonists were set to learn how the plants had been defeated originally, centuries before. Their path led them to a void dragon, a living weapon that was artificially created by other dragons. It had been betrayed and forced into exile after it destroyed the plants and the threat they posed. This dragon was a horrific creature, and the GM had designed this encounter as an opportunity for values clarification. The use of its magic required the consumption of life, and the intention was to prompt players to determine what their characters would be willing to sacrifice to save the world. The GM, role-playing the void dragon in a low, raspy tone, said, "Why should I help you? I am alone. The last of my kind with no family and no friends. Why should I save a world that has betrayed me?" One of the players leaned forward and said "That's just like me. I'm also alone and I have no friends. It's really hard." This was a profound moment of narrative transference for the player, as they saw their own lived experience of solitude and feelings of betrayal in the void dragon. As a response to this emergent moment, the GM shifted the encounter from one focused on values clarification to one focused on empathy and restitution. The void dragon became a sympathetic figure that the player sought to help, and in doing so they were able to validate their own lived experience. The player became a maternal figure to the void dragon, offering guidance and support as the void dragon learned to trust others and venture out into a sometimes harsh and unforgiving world.

Play-Based

While narrative transference can occur through a variety of narrative media, the Game to Grow Method utilizes the structure of TTRPGs to achieve these ends. It is important to note that the structure of TTRPGs is utilized not simply to provide systems of feedback and rewards, but to cultivate a sense of authentic relational social play into the narrative experience. The incorporation of play prompts participants to be immersed into the therapeutic experience, supports their growth, and instills a desire to continue. Dr. Stuart Brown (2010) defines play as having the following qualities: It is apparently purposeless, voluntary in nature, provides enjoyment, causes a suspension of sense of time, prompts a suspension of self-consciousness, has improvisational potential, and produces a desire to keep doing it. These aspects of play are each components of the Game to Grow Method. The unique, liminal qualities of the playspace created in TA-RPG make it a rich place for personal growth.

The Game to Grow Method utilizes TTRPGs to achieve its playful goals, but it should not be confused with "gamification" of therapy. Gamification is often described as the use of game mechanics in non-recreational environments to enhance motivation, concentration, effort, commitment, and other positive values common to all games (Fiuza-Fernández et al., 2022). Frequently, the game mechanics incorporated in gamification are leveraged to make something that is functionally uninteresting or otherwise undesirable more tolerable by injecting an extrinsic reward, such as victory points or achievements. While TA-RPG is generally open to gamification (e.g., a therapist could provide game-based incentives in a TTRPG as rewards for skill practice or completed homework), extrinsic rewards have been shown to reduce engagement and decrease the intrinsic value of participation in an activity (Kohn, 2018). The Game to Grow Method prioritizes leveraging the intrinsic motivations and inherent rewards of play over game-based extrinsic rewards.

Though TA-RPGs are focused on participant goals, they can often be described as a covert therapy. While the experience may at times be challenging and participants will likely feel uncomfortable as they progress toward therapeutic outcomes, the "voluntary" and "apparently purposeless" nature of TA-RPGs makes it feel less like "work." As mentioned in stories throughout this text, many of the individuals seen by the authors in TA-RPG groups have been fatigued by traditional therapy methods and found the experience of a play-based alternative to be a welcome change. They had experienced directive groups in which they felt they were expected to reveal their struggles or talk about their feelings with strangers. The play of TA-RPG supports participants to actually enjoy their therapeutic experience. Participants will still be able to benefit from their experiences, even if the work being done is not directed overtly by a therapist.

It may be difficult for TA-RPG facilitators to engage in intentional therapeutic interventions that may appear ostensibly "purposeless" to outsiders. Using the session design elements in Chapter 10, and the documentation guidelines in Chapter 13, the facilitator should always be able to identify the intention behind the intervention and progress toward goals even while engaging in the covert therapy of TA-RPG. Additionally, a required treatment can still feel "voluntary" through the way the facilitator respects participants' individual autonomy as they run the session. Instead of using coercive or manipulative tactics to correct behavior (methods that may be familiar and expected from therapy-fatigued participants), TA-RPG facilitators accept and welcome participant input with genuine curiosity. It will also be important for TA-RPG facilitators to remember that a shared group experience of play will support many participants in their goals. For many participants, the positive social experience will serve as behavioral activation, and will support their social practice. The session should feel like an opportunity to practice authentic social relationships because it should actually be an opportunity to practice authentic social relationships.

The TA-RPG experience should be absorbing, allowing participants to be fully present in the process and reduce their self-consciousness. Many well-run TA-RPG sessions will end with a collective groan from the participants as they are surprised that the session is "already over." This level of playful engagement can be described as a state of flow (Nakamura & Csikszentmihalyi, 2014). When participants are engaged in play and absorbed into the activity, they reduce their anxiety and any need to perform perfectly. The improvisational potential in a playful TA-RPG experience helps participants to be more curious about possibilities and open to discoveries. When participants play in this way, they are more willing to try new things, take risks, and experience the rewards of unpredictable outcomes.

As play is self-motivating and elicits a desire to continue participating, it is a crucial aspect to the Game to Grow Method. This continuation desire encourages continued attendance from individuals who may be treatment fatigued or otherwise have low interest in participation in a social activity. Enjoyment has been cited by child, adolescent, and adult learners as important for increasing motivation, engagement with material, and retention of information (Ares & Gorrell, 2002, Lucardie, 2014).

TA-RPG features imaginative narrative play, which allows the play to function in a simulated environment of "make-believe." While participants are unlikely to encounter the exact scenarios they encounter in the game (such as convincing an elf baker/wizard to give them the keys to the magic bakery's secret basement), the skills participants use in such situations will translate to real-world scenarios. For example, participants may use the lessons of self-advocacy to ask a teacher or boss for support, or to negotiate roles for a group project. Indeed, skills taught and practiced in simulated environments translate to the real world, and are commonly used in medicine (Alinier et al., 2006, Cook et al., 2011, Okuda et al., 2008, Sturm et al., 2008), sport (Fadde & Zaichkowsky, 2018), and flight training (De Winter et al., 2012; Hays et al., 1992).

This narrative, make-believe, playspace has additional qualities that will be important for TA-RPG facilitators to recognize and reinforce. The playspace created in TA-RPG is separated from the real world through the group acknowledgment of the activity, what can be described as a "magic circle" (Huizinga, 1955). This designation of an alternative space to real-world interactions allows participants to engage in the experience as players with a collective understanding that their interactions will be outside of the norms of everyday life. For example, in normal life, an individual may be considered rude or selfish if they thwart the intentions of another person, but in the "magic circle" of a game, they may be encouraged, recognized, and celebrated for this type of interaction. Likewise, when the game is over, the players return to their everyday expectations of each other. The check-in and check-out participation structures outlined in Chapter 10 are designed to support the group recognition of a designated "magic circle" of play, supporting participants to try new behaviors and interaction styles in the playspace.

The "magic circle" of TTRPGs is not entirely sealed off from real life. TTRPGs invite participants to simultaneously be their character and *not* their character. They are both the player at the table and the fictional character they portray, and while they are both, they are also neither. This aspect of the TTRPG playspace has been described as a "liminal space" (Bowman, 2010). This "betwixt and between" quality of the TTRPG is important for TA-RPGs because it allows for deconstruction and reconstruction of identity similar to a ritual or rite of passage. When participants enter into the playspace, they escape from their everyday circumstances to an environment unburdened by the norms and defined power structures of reality. In doing so, they can deconstruct their own identity (and that of their character). In the liminal playspace, they can reflect on the aspects of their character and their own identity and re-integrate aspects into a new self-concept. The liminal quality of this intervention is also exemplified in the emphasis on transition rituals (see Chapter 10), and in how the therapeutic GM guides participants to connect with and reflect on in-game scenarios both as themselves and as their characters (see Chapter 10).

Sometimes engaging in playful TA-RPG will require abandoning adherence to the specific rules of the game system. If the GM understands the structured rules of the game as the container that enables therapeutic play—the means to the end—they will be more flexible in their facilitation style and more open to the cultivation of play. As Brown mentions, "Play is a state of mind, rather than an activity" (p. 60). The therapeutic GM will need a sense of playfulness to meaningfully guide the play experience for participants and to serve as an important model to participants who may not have a personal history of play (referred to by Brown as a "play deficit"). For more details on the value of playfulness in TA-RPG facilitators, see SPARK in Chapter 12.

A Tale From the Real-World Table

Two adolescent players in a youth social flourishing group struggled to collaborate. One was a meticulous planner and the other was quick to act without thinking. Their dispositions were reflected in the characters they portrayed and in the way they interacted as players around the table. Seemingly every time the players were presented with an in-game obstacle that prompted their collaboration, they would argue unproductively about how to proceed, often slowing the game to a crawl and reducing the enjoyment for all involved. In a "gamified" skills-instruction model, the GM may have stopped the game (i.e., a mild punishment), taught interpersonal skills, and then provided incentives for their execution (i.e., extrinsic rewards). Leveraging the Game to Grow Method, the GM reflected the scenario into the playspace. On their journey to overthrow a corrupt king, the players' characters encountered a stubborn two-headed monster they sought to recruit to assist them in their efforts to attack the corrupt king's castle. The GM role-played the monster by holding his hands up and puppeteering the two heads, using a unique and silly voice for each. When the players role-played the interactions with the monster, they realized that the monster's two heads mirrored their own interaction style: One was a hot-headed improviser and the other was prone to anxiously overthink. The players laughed sheepishly as they recognized their own interpersonal struggles in the make-believe of the game. The GM then cartoonishly puppeteered the monster punching itself in the face, and the players laughed out loud at how their argumentative styles prevented their progress. The players recognized their own disposition in the respective monster head and gave it the advice that they needed to hear. The overplanner told his corresponding monster head that it would need to take some risks to accomplish goals, and the impulsive player instructed his corresponding monster head that sometimes it would need to pause and reflect before acting. These interactions were occurring in the "magic circle" of the game, but they reflected their lived experience and needs. Over time the two players learned to play together, and while they would often continue to disagree, they were able to navigate and negotiate their conflicts with a spirit of camaraderie. When the two players would argue during the check-in process or the check-out rituals, the GM would hold his hands up to mimic the two monster heads fighting, and the reference would playfully remind the players of their in-game journey. None of the meaningful interactions were based on the rules of the game system, but were made possible only in the playspace and enhanced by the collective engagement in true play.

Aesthetically Distanced

In many TTRPGs, players have a single character to portray. They often make intentional decisions for the character's unique skills and abilities, and create a unique personality for their character. As discussed earlier, there is a wealth of opportunity for players to experience transference and projection in the process of creating and portraying a character in a TTRPG, and the liminal playspace allows for players to identify with their character in multiple ways. At times, players will conceptualize their character as a game avatar that they control in a social activity. At other times, they will speak in the first person about their character and feel profound emotional resonance. As players play a TTRPG, the amount to which they emotionally and cognitively relate with a character can vary, and this spectrum of player/character identification is called aesthetic distance.

The concept of aesthetic distance comes from the writings of Edward Bullough (1912), wherein he describes the range of experiences one can have with art, delineating a range of "under-distance" to "over-distance." When a piece of art is too "close," it can cause an unpleasant overwhelming emotional state, and when it is too "distanced," it becomes difficult to enjoy. There is an optimal distance that allows the viewer to both experience the emotional resonance of the piece and not be overwhelmed by it. He illustrates the concept using an allegorical explanation of a sailor at sea looking at a fog in the distance. If the fog is too close to the sailor, it would be dangerous and terrifying. At an increased distance, the sailor would only notice the "objective" features of the fog, but at an optimal aesthetic distance the sailor would be able to experience the fog as an enjoyable aesthetic experience.

Translated to TA-RPG, the concept of aesthetic distance informs the ways a player identifies with their character. When a player is disconnected from the character, possibly to the point of viewing them as a list of mechanics on a sheet of paper, the participant is considered "over-distanced" from the character. In that moment, they do not have an emotional connection to the character, and are no longer experiencing the story through the character but as a player in an objective experience. When a participant is so closely connected with a character that they identify with their character's triumphs and disasters, experiencing the character's emotional landscape as their own, they are "under-distanced" from their character. Under-distanced players may struggle to regulate their emotions when exciting or upsetting events happen with their character.

The range of aesthetic distance occurs naturally in TTRPGs. Players will often vary in their aesthetic distance as a reflection of their general play style (some are more comfortable with and may prefer closer aesthetic distance), and players may individually experience close and far aesthetic distance over the course of a single session depending on the narrative transference of the particular story moment and the player's immersion in the play. Some players will regularly use the first person to declare their character's actions (i.e., they have a "close aesthetic distance") and express their character's emotions, while others use the third person to narrate their character's actions with a flatter affect (i.e., they have a "far aesthetic distance").

Understanding how a player relates to their character enables understanding of the narrative transference present in the TA-RPG playspace, and recognizing their degree of aesthetic distance allows the TA-RPG facilitator to guide the player's insight and acquisition of skills. The therapeutic GM's intentional guidance of the player's aesthetic distance assists them in expanding aesthetic distance to externalize their challenges onto their character and gain insight, or reducing aesthetic distance to internalize the successes of their character as their own. For more details on this concept, see "character types" in Chapter 8 and "Pronouns for Aesthetic Distance" in Chapter 11.

A Tale From the Real-World Table

A group of players were gathering for an initial session, and many had brought their own characters that had not yet been seen by the GM. The GM narrated the opening encounter: All of the players' characters entered a secure building and were required to place any weapons or magical items into a magically sealed chest. As the characters met their first non-player character (NPC), skeletons suddenly burst through the walls and the floors and began to threaten the inhabitants of the secure building. This encounter was designed to encourage the players' creative problem solving, and the GM asked each player, in turn order, what their character would do to protect themselves and the other inhabitants of the building against the onslaught of undead. One player held up his hands and declared: "I summon my weapons to myself!" He had designed his character with runic tattoos on his forearms that would magically teleport his two swords to his hands. This player was experiencing a close aesthetic distance, as evidenced by his use of the first person and raised hands. The GM responded, "Your weapons are sealed in a magical chest. They don't teleport to you." The player became dysregulated. He looked at his forearms as if they would have his character's tattoos across them, and in short breaths said "No! I made my character to summon my weapons to myself!" In response to this under-distance, the GM said, "*Your character* expected those weapons to show up. The skeletons are attacking and *he* wanted those weapons to appear in *his* hands but they didn't. *He's really* mad. What does *he* do next?" Through the use of pronouns, the GM extended the player's aesthetic distance, allowing the player to consider the character as separate from himself. The player's display of angry affect shifted to a flat, curious affect. He paused for a moment and then declared in the third person, "He rips the arms off the skeleton and beats them with their own arms!" Seeing that the player was now emotionally regulated and that he had increased his aesthetic distance with his character, the GM wanted to close the aesthetic distance again and replied enthusiastically, "Yes! You do! You were mad but you pushed through! You throttle the skeleton with its own arms!" The GM's guidance back toward first-person language assisted the player to internalize and identify with the experience of re-regulating after a setback and their character's triumph over the skeleton.

Developmental

A core principle of the Game to Grow Method is that it is not a manualized, one-size-fits-all treatment. The model is designed to facilitate growth consistent with the participant's values and goals. It respects and appreciates participants' individual differences in capacity and development, both holistically and in a session-to-session context. TA-RPGs should be accessible to a broad range of participants, sometimes even together in diverse groups. TA-RPG facilitators are expected to plan sessions to meet individuals' global, developmental needs, as well as to adjust accordingly to the individual needs that manifest that day.

The developmental approach in the Game to Grow Method is a lifespan approach, with an acknowledgment that an individual's daily capacities may change based on internal and external contexts (e.g., their emotional state and the supports they are provided). The DIR/Floortime model (a key inspiration for the Core Capacities, see Chapter 8) is based on, and named for, a developmental and relational approach that respects individual differences (Wieder & Greenspan, 2006; Mercer, 2017). Creating a collaborative and respectful treatment environment is also a core component of many approaches that are compatible with the Game to Grow Method, such as Acceptance and Commitment Therapy (ACT), Humanistic, and Interpersonal approaches (Cooper, 2007; Wampold, 2015; Mallinckrodt, 2010).

When considering a participant's current capacities, both state and trait influences should be considered. Trait influences may be internal to the participant or based on prior experiences and context. For example, a participant's cognitive development will impact their ability to perspective take and use deductive reasoning. This is an internal influence that will change over time as the participant develops, but will remain fairly static on a day-to-day basis. In contrast, if a participant has a history of abusive interpersonal relationships, they may struggle to develop appropriate trust in current relationships as such trust development may not have been adaptive or rewarded in prior learning environments. Trait influences on development are not necessarily permanent, but may have a more persistent impact on a participant's capacity to connect with others.

State influences are immediate and short-term influences to a participant's internal experience, which can negatively impact their capacity to connect with others. Common negative influences can be identified using the acronym "HALT," which stands for hungry, angry (or other frustrated-type emotions), lonely (or other sad/disconnected emotions), and tired. When possible, these negative state influences should be addressed, such as by having snacks available for hungry participants. However, not all state influences can be adjusted in the moment, especially those related to emotions that were prompted by outside-of-session events. When state influences cannot be readily resolved, bringing awareness to the state in a supporting and accepting way can support the facilitator, the participant, and the group's ability to make space for the experience and have compassion for the potential impact on the participant's capacity to participate. State influences that support a participant's expression of a Core Capacity are also important to accommodate. This can include support from other players, predictability of the situation, or the experience of success in or out of the game.

Regarding developmental foundations, the primary focus of the Game to Grow Method is on supporting individuals in areas related to their goals and the Core Capacities. Notably, participants are likewise developing competencies related to TTRPGs as they participate in their particular group. TA-RPG facilitators who use a developmental approach to participants' growth in their Core Capacities, as well as their capacity to engage in TTRPGs and game-related goals, will be able to more completely provide an opportunity for all participants to flourish.

In practice, a developmental approach to TA-RPGs requires facilitators to choose and adjust a game system to meet the developmental needs of participants (see "choosing a game system" in Chapter 6). To specifically support their players' ability to participate and benefit from the experience, facilitators plan and adjust the performance expectations (e.g., rolling dice and adding numbers mentally), the game difficulty (e.g., the challenge level of a combat encounter with monsters), and the game content (e.g., include a talking wolf to specifically engage a player with a special interest in canines). TA-RPG facilitators utilizing pre-written modules will likely need to adjust them significantly.

TA-RPG facilitators can adjust game content for individual players and for groups based on their developmental capacities. Depending on the stage of group development (see Chapter 9), the performance expectations, game difficulty, and game content can be tailored to the needs of the group. A group that is newly formed and struggling to work together may benefit from a simpler challenge, whereas one that has been working together collaboratively for an extended time period may thrive with a complex challenge. When groups are presented with a complex challenge, individual group members can be challenged at their individual level (e.g., some players may be challenged to speak as their character, while others may be asked to narrate their character's actions), while entire groups can be challenged simultaneously (e.g., working together to solve a puzzle that requires full group participation and communication).

A Tale From the Real-World Table

The player characters in a three-player adolescent group were on a large passenger ship, which was described to the players as being similar to a ferry from the Washington State transit system that was familiar to the players' real-world experience. The ship was headed toward calamity—a giant waterfall. They decided they would redirect the ship by secretly breaking into the wheelhouse, ensuring the other passengers were not alerted. The group consisted of three players: Two of the players were familiar with each other and TTRPGs, having played in the same TA-RPG group for several years. The third player was new to the group, new to TTRPGs, and had some intellectual disabilities that resulted in a need for significantly more support to participate. The group collectively decided that the newer player would cause a distraction while the experienced players sought entry to the wheelhouse. The GM understood the developmental discrepancies between the participants, and he set the participation challenges accordingly. The two experienced players were challenged to roll dice and use their characters' skills and abilities to collaboratively find entry to the locked wheelhouse. For them, this encounter was aligned to their goals of clear and effective communication and logical sequencing. The GM adjusted the challenge differently for the newer player. Recognizing the player's anxiety (a state influence) as a new player, as well as the developmental struggles with logical sequencing (a trait influence) the GM offered a wide invitation for input: "What do you want to do to create a distraction?" The new player suggested, "I'm going to make it a birthday party." He announced that he would get all of the passengers to sing happy birthday to someone on the ship. Instead of rolling any dice to determine how successful he would be at this endeavor, the GM asked, "Which person do you want to sing to? A younger person or an older person?" The player said, "An old lady."

"How many candles will you put on her cake?"

"One hundred!"

"You start handing streamers and decorations to everyone to help decorate the ship, then you emerge from the ship's galley with a cake that is so bright with all those candles that everyone looks at you in surprise. The old lady has a big smile on her face and says, 'You remembered my 100th birthday!' "

The GM then led the group of players in singing happy birthday to the "old lady" NPC, role-played by the GM as tearing up at the kindness of the new player's character. While the GM enacted the birthday party, he would periodically pause and shift the group's attention back to the players working to gain entry to the secured wheelhouse, offering them extra mechanical advantages based on the success of the birthday party distraction, leading the entire group to successfully redirect the ship and save the passengers.

The GM had adjusted the encounter to the individual developmental needs of the participants, shifting the performance expectations, encounter difficulty, and in-game content to meet their trait and state needs. At the end of the session, the players all celebrated their shared moment of triumph, and the new player received several compliments about his spontaneity and creative thinking. Such moments, over time and with repetition, helped the group continue to collaborate and play together. The newer player became more confident in their role as both a TTRPG player and a member of the group.

Scaffolded

While the developmental aspect of the Game to Grow Method instructs TA-RPG facilitators to design encounters to meet the state and trait needs of the players, it also recognizes that the facilitator can provide appropriate guidance and support to help participants learn and grow during the gameplay itself. This guidance and support is known as "scaffolding." One of the first uses of this term in a learning context was in a manuscript that identified the strategies of parents who successfully supported their children in completing challenging tasks (Wood et al., 1976). With guidance and support from a more experienced peer or a mentor, an individual has a higher capacity for growth. Effective scaffolding can involve modeling the task, helping to break the task into manageable pieces, aid in identifying crucial features, as well as support with maintaining attention and motivation on the task (Bruner, 1978). The concepts and theory of scaffolding are built within and commonly referenced with Vygotsky's work on the "zone of proximal development." Vygotsky argued that individual learning is heavily influenced by society and relationships, and when learning, support from a more skilled partner can increase a learner's capacity (Vygotsky, 1978). The theoretical place between actions a participant can do successfully without aid and actions a learner can accomplish with support is their "zone of proximal development," and scaffolding is a term used to describe the guidance and support to help a learner achieve more than they could accomplish alone.

Scaffolding methods are commonly used in educational settings to improve learning and create optimal levels of difficulty (Kim et al., 2018; Sanders & Welk, 2005). This principle can be translated to TA-RPGs, as therapeutic GMs are responsible for facilitating growth in their participants. The word "facilitator" comes from the Latin roots "Facilis," meaning "easy to do," and "ator," meaning a person or thing that performs an action. A TA-RPG facilitator is the one who provides the guidance and support (i.e., the scaffolding) that makes it easier for participants to engage in the experience and supports their growth.

TA-RPGs have ample scaffolding opportunities to support participants, through manipulation of the fantasy environment or narrative, communication with NPCs or the facilitator, and feedback from other participants or player characters. Because TTRPGs are typically a fantasy storytelling game, the facilitator's control over the environment, monsters, and NPCs provides multiple avenues for the facilitator to increase or decrease the difficulty of scenarios and add in supplemental guidance and support.

Scaffolding in TA-RPG can take many forms depending on the new skill or behavior being supported, including providing unconditional positive regard, re-framing situations, removing obstacles, reducing difficulty, and providing guidance through teaching, encouragement, reinforcement, feedback, and coaching. Each of these supports is leveraged to allow participants to fully engage in the opportunity for growth.

It is the facilitator's responsibility to create a safe and welcoming space where mistakes can be made. The facilitator's expression of unconditional positive regard will help create an environment where participants feel safe to try out identities, make mistakes, and practice (and fail at) new skills. This particular scaffolding does not mean that participants will always be comfortable. Growth is often uncomfortable. It is the facilitator's responsibility to create a safe and welcoming space to be uncomfortable and grow. Unconditional positive regard does not mean that facilitators will like or agree with all of a participant's behaviors, but instead are accepting and approving of the participants themselves. TA-RPG facilitators will show unconditional positive regard by expressing a compassionate understanding that participants will make mistakes, and that they have the capacity to learn from them.

Another scaffolding technique is to re-frame challenging situations, which is optimally supported by unconditional positive regard. Because the TA-RPG facilitator narrates the outcomes of character actions, they have the ability to attribute positive attributes to failures (e.g., a GM can describe the character's heroic resolve and perseverance after a setback). Doing so provides the participant the support they may need to recognize the value in their struggle. Similarly, a TA-RPG facilitator can invite a player to describe the outcomes of their character's unsuccessful actions, extending a sense of agency around their failure. If they can find joy in the narrative externalization of their character's failure, they may be able to look at it with a fresh perspective and see failure as an opportunity, instead of a setback. Through failure, one gains invaluable data, which can be used to calibrate behavior associated with future attempts.

TA-RPG facilitators can also re-frame a player's antagonistic or maladaptive action by attributing positive intent. Using functional analysis (see Chapter 8), the facilitator can identify what need a participant is attempting to meet through their expression of maladaptive behavior. Once identified, the facilitator can provide another opportunity to achieve that need, often while encouraging a more adaptive approach. A participant whose character engages in destructive in-game behavior that frustrates other group members (e.g., igniting a fire in a town the protagonists are working to save from monsters) may benefit from a facilitator attributing a positive intent (e.g., causing a distraction to draw the monsters away from the other characters). The GM may assume that the original intent of the destructive behavior was to gain attention (albeit negative) from the fellow players, and by reframing the intent as helpful they show the player a more prosocial way to get that attention. Doing so may help them learn new ways to meet their needs.

Scaffolding in TA-RPG may also include removing barriers to player participation. These barriers should be removed whenever possible through developmental session design, but should also be removed as unexpected situations emerge. The need for accessibility supports, for example, may not be directly shared by participants. However, such support should be explicitly available for participants to use. Additionally, if a participant has low stamina for social interaction, full participation in the check-in process may become a barrier to the participant's engagement in the gameplay portion of the session. In such cases, the player may benefit from removing the expectation of their full participation and allow them to give a short answer without pressure to elaborate.

Because GMs determine in-game difficulty and the success criteria for character actions, they can support growth by adjusting the difficulty of specific in-game encounters. Similar to the ways encounters can be designed developmentally, GMs can adjust both the performance expectations and in-game difficulty of an encounter to support player growth. A risk-averse player who decides their character will take an appropriate risk may benefit from a feeling of success. Where a GM might otherwise determine a static success criteria (i.e., a specific number a player would need to roll on their dice), a TA-RPG facilitator would lower the requirement for success to allow the player to experience the triumph. When providing scaffolding by reducing difficulty, it is important that the facilitator adjusts the challenge to support the participant in completing the act, as opposed to removing the challenge completely or completing the act for them.

Though scaffolding is often talked about in conjunction with supports that decrease the level of stress or difficulty of a scenario, increasing difficulty can also serve to scaffold an individual's skills. Research has shown that variable simulated pressure helps skills translate more effectively to real-world situations (Low et al., 2020). If a participant feels comfortable advocating for themselves or other participants in low-stress situations, increasing the stress of the situation appropriately can provide space for the participant to increase their advocacy skills in higher stress situations. Variability of situation and difficulty can help further cement an individual's confidence and ability to flexibly apply skills in a variety of situations.

The TA-RPG facilitator can also scaffold player growth by providing direct support for capacity development. They can provide information, encouragement, reinforcement, feedback, and opportunities to try again (see "Three Dimensions of Capacity Building" in Chapter 8). These scaffolds can occur through the facilitator, through an NPC, or through additional in-game events.

Finally, facilitators should maintain awareness of contextual factors that may impact the participant's demonstration of the supported skill, such as the behavior of other participants, the participant's (or their character's) current goals, or the time left in session. For example, if a participant is dysregulated, they are unlikely to be able to learn or display a challenging skill as effectively as when they are regulated (Fraser et al., 2012). Slowing down the speed of the encounter, reducing the intensity of communication, or changing the focus from the participant to their character are some ways to support regulation for participants and cultivate an environment conducive to learning.

A Tale From the Real-World Table

It was the fourth TA-RPG session of a six-person group for veterans with severe mental illness diagnoses. The group had been exploring a labyrinthine mine, hoping to find a lost treasure that would grant the party riches, glory, and possible immortality. However, only two of the six players were able to attend the group that particular day. One of the presenting players had treatment goals of becoming more assertive and improving their self-esteem, while the other player aimed to become more flexible and creative. Both players had been comfortably passive during previous sessions, happy to defer to other players to make decisions for choices that impacted the entire party, such as which direction to move or strategy to use when overcoming obstacles. The GM confirmed the other players would be absent and asked the two remaining players what they wanted to do. One of the players voiced their concern that the most vocal and experienced player was not present to provide the guidance and leadership they had become accustomed to. The other player agreed and said, "I want to play today. I looked forward to today all week, but I'm afraid we're going to get ourselves killed without the others." The GM acknowledged the player's plight and the perceived danger of their two characters continuing alone. The GM knew the players would benefit from external support and chose to scaffold the players through the use of an NPC to model, prompt, and reinforce behaviors associated with their goals. Through the NPC that the group brought with them into the mine, the GM said, "Do you want to take a risk? I know it is dangerous, but I think this could be an opportunity to see what we can do on our own. I think you two are more capable than you realize." After a moment of silence, the two players looked at each other and smiled. "If you were looking forward to playing, I think we should play. I trust you and if we move carefully, I think we could impress the others." The two spent the session navigating the maze-like interior of the mine, sneaking past monsters, solving puzzles, and safely triggering or disarming traps. Throughout the session, the GM used the NPC to prompt behaviors aligned with the players' treatment goals. At first, the GM scaffolded the player's development by using the NPC to model assertive behavior and flexibility, voicing simple solutions to simple problems and expressing their willingness to try new things and make mistakes if it helped their companions. With time, the players became more comfortable expressing simple ideas, but hesitated to voice their solutions to more complex problems. In such moments, the NPC would voice their own terrible ideas, designed to be bad enough to prompt the players to disagree. The GM's use of the NPC scaffolded players to practice asserting their dissent and brainstorming alternative, safer solutions. When players would take a risk by sharing their ideas or overcoming an obstacle, the NPC would respond with approval and gratitude for their creativity and bravery. Further, the GM was mindful to reduce performance expectations and difficulty during such moments to support confidence and self-esteem. At the end of the session, one of the players voiced "We did better than I expected. Maybe we are more capable than I thought." The following week, these players proudly expressed their victories to the other group members. Their fellow group members expressed a desire to help them reach their goals, requesting they lead the party more frequently and pausing to ask them for their opinions before making decisions as a group. Over the next several sessions, these two players continued to build confidence in themselves and their leadership abilities. The GM continued to scaffold these players toward their goals, gradually increasing the stress of encounters to match their developing skills. At the end of this TA-RPG group, one of these two players applied for and was offered a job that required communication and leadership skills, which they directly attributed to the scaffolding they received in the group. They shared that the group helped them build confidence in themselves, worry less about other people's perceptions of them, and become more comfortable stepping out of their comfort zone.

Relational

Relationships are a core aspect of the Game to Grow Method. The relational aspect refers to the function of relationships in the treatment itself, as well as the importance placed on relationships as a goal and an outcome to be celebrated. To support participants' social flourishing, TA-RPG facilitators work to support participants' capacity to meaningfully connect with others in a way that is consistent with their values. As such, the relationships built in TA-RPG groups are core to that foundation and goal.

Consistent with the wide body of literature supporting the importance of common factors such as alliance, empathy, expectations, and cultural adaptation, the relationships within the groups are seen as paramount to support insight, growth, and change for participants (Wampold, 2015). Similar to other therapy groups, TA-RPG groups feature relationships between facilitator and participant, as well as relationships between participants. Because TA-RPGs are based on shared narrative role-play in which players are guided to identify with and grow through their characters, TA-RPG groups will also feature relationships between characters in the story. While relationships with these fictional characters will be different from those participants have with the facilitator or their peers around the table, these characters can provide further opportunities for growth and insight. Though there are a variety of relationships in TA-RPG, both real and fictional, core tenets of functional relationships, such as mutual respect, perspective taking, and boundaries, are present across these relationships.

As mentioned previously, the facilitator's guidance and support can be instrumental in cultivating participant insight, as well as in creating a sense of group safety and trust. The strength of the relationship between facilitator and the group members is especially important during initial group formation, as members begin to learn the structure and expectations of the group. As the participants become more established, the facilitator's unconditional positive regard provides them the safety to make mistakes, share personal reflections, and ask for help.

The impact of peer relationships and the value of the cohort in TA-RPGs groups are hard to overestimate. Within group psychotherapy, levels of group cohesion are positively correlated with treatment outcome (Burlingame et al., 2011). Additionally, group cohesion elements such as group functioning, bonding, and encouragement positively correlate with outcomes in groups with youth (Shechtman & Leichtentritt, 2010). The interpersonal learning within TA-RPGs is often more experiential and immediate than scripted or rote learning. Further, focus on relationships in the group allows for opportunities to practice healthy communication strategies. The strength of relationships in the group empowers participants to engage in more challenging interpersonal interactions, and create a strong base for repair when ruptures and misunderstandings occur.

For adolescents and adults, peer modeling and referencing is developmentally appropriate, meaning that participants should be referring to each other, not just the facilitator, as they are making social decisions. Further, for these groups, feedback from other participants is often more powerful than feedback from the facilitator, as there can be a perception that the facilitator "has to" be nice, while peers are under no such edict.

Similar to other group interventions, TA-RPGs rely on the social microcosm, which is a term used to describe the interflow of behaviors between participants' lives inside and outside of a group. Participants replicate their real-world interpersonal behaviors in group, and as they learn new behaviors in group, they will start to use these behaviors outside of group. Though there may be confidentiality around topics discussed in the group, there is no such confidentiality around learned behaviors.

Leveraging narrative transference and aesthetic distance, the relationships between the characters portrayed by the players and the NPCs in the story can be powerful vectors for insight and growth. Participants may not have a history of rewarding social experiences with strangers, and may be more comfortable interacting socially as their character with an NPC portrayed by the GM. This may be an approachable "entry point" when learning to develop relationships among participants who may find interacting directly with other participants to be too dysregulating. The facilitator can provide scaffolding to the interactions as appropriate to allow for the player to learn effective interpersonal strategies. For example, an NPC who engages in annoying behavior may prompt a valuable opportunity to practice giving feedback and setting boundaries.

Similarly, supporting players to interact through their characters allows for externalization of thoughts, feelings, and behaviors. Through externalization, participants can observe and reflect on both adaptive and maladaptive relational patterns, experimenting safely with relational cause and effect. For example, a player may role-play an overly aggressive character while working to develop social confidence, gaining insight into the pros and cons of aggressive behavior. If another player explains how it negatively impacts their character, the player can gain valuable insight without personal feelings of failure. With time, their character can use this insight to evolve into a more prosocial, assertive character with the confidence to ensure their needs are more consistently met.

A Tale From the Real-World Table

Two players in a four-person group for emerging adults had been arguing in character as a way to externalize their interpersonal conflict. In real life, they seemed to enjoy each other's company, laughing together during sessions and sharing in the triumphs of the story, but would also occasionally experience conflicts they did not have the tools to address directly. Both would playfully insult or demean each other in character, and occasionally thwart the others' in-game strategies. The GM saw this as a valuable opportunity to reflect on their relationship through the externalization of their conflict onto their characters. The GM asked the two of them what was happening in their character's relationships. "What's going on between the two of them?" The players each reflected that their characters were frustrated with the other in a way that perfectly mirrored the conflicts experienced by the two players at the table. One player mentioned that the other player's character always thought they knew best and never listened to anyone else's ideas. The second player replied, "*You* never listen to *my character's* ideas!"

The GM inquired to the two of them, "What should happen in the story that will help your characters work through their conflict?" The players decided that their characters would not be able to talk it over and that they would fight each other. Reflecting back to the players that the characters were allies who had worked together for years, the GM facilitated their conflict with a narrative tone of tragedy. When one of the players cast a powerful spell that seriously injured the other, the players paused after the GM's somber description. One player said, "I rush over to her and I say 'I'm so sorry! I didn't mean to hurt you!'" The other player, roleplaying their injured character, said "No, I'm sorry."

With minimal guidance from the GM, the two players then roleplayed a series of apologies (all in character) about how they had interacted and how they would try to listen to each other more. They each mentioned how much their relationship meant to them and how they would work to not take it for granted. While the communication between the two individuals was in-character, the substance of their conversation was directed at each other. They were mutually acknowledging the importance of their relationship and working through their conflict in the safety of the playspace. The two players' ability to externalize their relational conflict onto their characters allowed them to give and receive necessary feedback and feel the authentic value of their personal connection.

References

Alinier, G., Hunt, B., Gordon, R., & Harwood, C. (2006). Effectiveness of intermediate-fidelity simulation training technology in undergraduate nursing education. *Journal of Advanced Nursing, 54*(3), 359–369. https://doi.org/10.1111/j.1365-2648.2006.03810.x

American Psychological Association. (n.d.). *APA dictionary of psychology*. Retrieved from https://dictionary.apa.org/transference

Ares, N., & Gorrell, J. (2002). Middle school students' understanding of meaningful learning and engaging classroom activities. *Journal of Research in Childhood Education, 16*(2), 263–277. https://doi.org/10.1080/02568540209594989

Bowman, S. L. (2010). *The functions of role-playing games: How participants create community, solve problems and explore identity*. McFarland & Co.

Brown, S. (2010). *Play: How it shapes the brain, opens the imagination, and invigorates the soul*. Avery.

Bruner, J. S. (1978). The role of dialogue in language acquisition. In A. Sinclair, R. Jarvella, & W. J. M. Levelt (Eds.), *The child's conception of language*. Springer-Verlag.

Bullough, E. (1912). 'Psychic Distance' as a factor in art and as an aesthetic principle. *British Journal of Psychology*. (5), 87–117.

Burlingame, G. M., McClendon, D. T., & Alonso, J. (2011). Cohesion in group therapy. *Psychotherapy, 48*(1), 34–42. https://doi.org/10.1037/a0022063

Cook, D. A., Hatala, R., Brydges, R., Zendejas, B., Szostek, J. H., Wang, A. T., . . . & Hamstra, S. J. (2011). Technology-enhanced simulation for health professions education: A systematic review and meta-analysis. *JAMA, 306*(9), 978–988. https://doi.org10.1001/jama.2011.1234

Cooper, M. (2007). Humanizing psychotherapy. *Journal of Contemporary Psychotherapy, 37*(1), 11–16. https://doi.org/10.1007/s10879-006-9029-6

De Winter, J. C., Dodou, D., & Mulder, M. (2012). Training effectiveness of whole body flight simulator motion: A comprehensive meta-analysis. *The International Journal of Aviation Psychology, 22*(2), 164–183. https://doi.org/10.1080/10508 414.2012.663247

Fadde, P. J., & Zaichkowsky, L. (2018). Training perceptual-cognitive skills in sports using technology. *Journal of Sport Psychology in Action, 9*(4), 239–248. https://doi.org/10.1080/21520704.2018.1509162

Fiuza-Fernández, A., Lomba-Portela, L., Soto-Carballo, J., & Pino-Juste, M. R. (2022). Study of the knowledge about gamification of degree in primary education students. *PLoS One, 17*(3), e0263107. https://doi.org/10.1371/journal.pone.0263107

Fraser, K., Ma, I., Teteris, E., Baxter, H., Wright, B., & McLaughlin, K. (2012). Emotion, cognitive load and learning outcomes during simulation training. *Medical Education, 46*(11), 1055–1062. https://doi.org/10.1111/j.1365-2923.2012.04355.x

Hays, R. T., Jacobs, J. W., Prince, C., & Salas, E. (1992). Flight simulator training effectiveness: A meta-analysis. *Military Psychology, 4*(2), 63–74. https://doi.org/10.1207/s15327876mp0402_1

Horton, D., & Wohl, R. R. (1956). Mass communication and para-social interaction: Observations on intimacy at a distance. *Psychiatry, 19*(3), 215–229. https://doi.org/10.1080/00332747.1956.11023049

Huizinga, J. (1955). *Homo Ludens: A study of the play-element in culture*. The Beacon Press.

Kim, N. J., Belland, B. R., & Axelrod, D. (2018). Scaffolding for optimal challenge in K-12 problem-based learning. *The Interdisciplinary Journal of Problem-based Learning, 13*(1), Article 3. https://doi.org/10.7771/1541-5015.1712

Kohn, A. (2018). *Punished by rewards*. Houghton Mifflin Harcourt Trade & Reference Publishers.

Low, W. R., Sandercock, G. R. H., Freeman, P., Winter, M. E., Butt, J., & Maynard, I. (2020). Pressure training for performance domains: A meta-analysis. *Sport, Exercise, and Performance Psychology, 10*(1), 149–163. https://doi.org/10.1037/spy0000202

Lucardie, D. (2014). The impact of fun and enjoyment on adult's learning. *Procedia - Social and Behavioral Sciences, 142*, 439–446. https://doi.org/10.1016/j.sbspro.2014.07.696

Mallinckrodt, B. (2010). The psychotherapy relationship as attachment: Evidence and implications. *Journal of Social and Personal Relationships, 27*(2), 262–270. https://doi.org/10.1177/0265407509360905

Mercer, J. (2017). Examining DIR/Floortime™ as a treatment for children with autism spectrum disorders: A review of research and theory. *Research on Social Work Practice, 27*(5), 625–635.

Nakamura, J., & Csikszentmihalyi, M. (2014). The concept of flow. In *Flow and the foundations of positive psychology*. Dordrecht: Springer. https://doi.org/10.1007/978-94-017-9088-8_16

Okuda, Y., Bond, W., Bonfante, G., McLaughlin, S., Spillane, L., Wang, E., . . . & Gordon, J. A. (2008). National growth in simulation training within emergency medicine residency programs, 2003–2008. *Academic Emergency Medicine, 15*(11), 1113–1116. https://doi.org/10.1111/j.1553-2712.2008.00195.x

Prasko, J., Diveky, T., Grambal, A., Kamaradova, D., Mozny, P., Sigmundova, Z., . . . & Vyskocilova, J. (2010). Transference and countertransference in cognitive behavioral therapy. *Biomedical Papers, 154*(3), 189–197.

Sanders, D., & Welk, D. S. (2005). Strategies to scaffold student learning: Applying Vygotsky's zone of proximal development. *Nurse Educator, 30*(5), 203–207.

Shechtman, Z., & Leichtentritt, J. (2010). The association of process with outcomes in child group therapy. *Psychotherapy Research, 20*(1), 8–21.

Sturm, L. P., Windsor, J. A., Cosman, P. H., Cregan, P., Hewett, P. J., & Maddern, G. J. (2008). A systematic review of skills transfer after surgical simulation training. *Annals of Surgery, 248*(2), 166–179. http://doi.org10.1097/SLA.0b013e318176bf24

Vygotsky, L. S. (1978). *Mind in society: The development of higher psychological processes* (M. Cole et al., Ed.). Harvard University Press.

Wampold, B. E. (2015). How important are the common factors in psychotherapy? An update. *World Psychiatry, 14*(3), 270–277.

Wieder, S., & Greenspan, S. I. (2006). Infant and Early Childhood Mental Health: The DIR model. In G. M. Foley & J. D. Hochman (Eds.), *Mental health in early intervention: Achieving unity in principles and practice* (pp. 175–189). Paul H. Brookes Publishing.

Wood, D., Bruner, J. S., & Ross, G. (1976). The role of tutoring in problem solving. *Child Psychology & Psychiatry & Allied Disciplines, 17*(2), 89–100. https://doi.org/10.1111/j.1469-7610.1976.tb00381.x

6

Choosing the Right Tabletop Role-Playing Game System for Your Therapeutically Applied Role-Playing Game Group

When facilitating a therapeutically applied role-playing game (TA-RPG) group, therapeutic game masters (GMs) must select a game system they will leverage for participant growth. When selecting a tabletop role-playing game (TTRPG) system, it is important to keep in mind that every TTRPG has opportunities for targeted and intentional growth, though the differences between the game systems are necessary to consider when selecting a game system for a particular group of individuals. The choice of which game to play is multifaceted, including the consideration of popularity, structural game design, system complexity, age-appropriateness, setting/genre, and personal taste.

Each TTRPG game system is a combination of rules that create the basic foundation for playing a game, a setting in which the game's story takes place. Dungeons & Dragons (D&D) is one popular system, so are Pathfinder, Shadowrun, Starfinder, Fiasco, Night Witches, and Vampire: The Masquerade. Each of these games, and many more, contain a setting or settings in which the game takes place (e.g., the mystical land of Toverus, the city of Waterdeep) and a genre (e.g., fantasy, science fiction, Victorian era historical fiction). They also contain a set of rules that help to define how the game is played. These rules detail structural aspects such as the roles and responsibilities of the players and any randomization tools, as well as finer details about how characters are created and how players make choices through their character. All of these games share one major thing in common: The goal is to tell an interesting and engaging collaborative story with contributions from all participants. When used as a therapeutic tool, the goals will go beyond the specific purpose of story creation for which the game is designed.

While this chapter will provide suggestions of different existing game systems, the GM should always make sure to be reasonably knowledgeable and aware of both the setting and game mechanics of any game that they select. In many situations, being comfortable enough with a game system and setting to be able to adjust the rules or setting (often spontaneously) can be much more valuable and impactful toward the

DOI: 10.4324/9781003281962-6

therapeutic outcomes for group members than the selection of a different game would be. There are many different game settings and systems to choose from, and the decision of which one is best for a specific treatment or group can seem overwhelming. However, one of the most important factors in selecting the right TTRPG for a group will always be the facilitator's comfort and familiarity with the selected game systems. Competence to run a multitude of game systems will provide greater flexibility when working with various populations, allowing facilitators to select games that best align with the skill level, engagement, or cultural expression of the members of the group.

Popularity

Among TTRPGs, Dungeons & Dragons stands out as the most popular and recognizable TTRPG in existence (Roll20, 2022). Its name alone evokes recognition, excitement, and sometimes infamy, even from those who have no experience or exposure to TTRPGs.

Parents, teachers, and therapists alike will often be familiar with the name D&D, creating an access point for new players. Players, who may not know anything about TTRPGs, have likely heard the name Dungeons & Dragons (often referred to as "D&D") through TV shows, movies, news articles, video games, and word of mouth. This popularity creates a unique and valuable comparison point for other game systems, which can be helpful when advocating for systems that utilize mechanics or settings that may be better suited to support the most auspicious growth-oriented play for a certain population. TA-RPG facilitators may run a multitude of different game systems, but consistently reference D&D as a way to compare and contrast game systems for new families and participants (e.g., "It is a role-playing game, like D&D, but in space").

The popularity of a game system provides additional support for participants, in the form of increased accessibility outside of the TA-RPG group. Many game stores around the world have recreational D&D groups that they run each week. Anecdotally, within the United States, it may be easier to find social groups playing D&D than it is for any other specific role-playing game. For groups focused on improving participants' number and quality of relationships and their capacity to connect with others, having the secondary benefit of building the knowledge and skill to participate in a social hobby can be invaluable. For those participants, TTRPGs become a tool that they can utilize in other parts of their life to build positive social relationships with other people on their own terms. Thus, there are distinct advantages to selecting the more popular option when making the choice between two different games systems.

There are other options for game systems that are rising in popularity. Notable mentions include Pathfinder and Starfinder, Call of Cthulhu, Shadowrun, Vampire: The Masquerade, and the Star Wars RPG.

The Role of the Game Master

Typically, TTPRGs feature asymmetric roles of play where one player acts as the GM. The GM describes scenes and sets the tone of the story while players choose the actions for their single character. This role is useful when using the game as a therapeutic tool, as it allows the therapist to be the GM and make intentional and meaningful changes to the story, setting, and outcomes. However, some TTRPGs forgo the role of GM, creating a scenario where all of the players at the table have the same level of power and input to impact the shared storytelling experience. Because these games have no GM, these story-focused games are often referred to as "GM-less games."

An exemplary GM-less game is Fiasco, a storytelling game inspired by popular stories of failed escapades and mischief gone awry. Fiasco focuses on dice rolls to determine the characters, content, and outcome of storytelling scenes, but provides the space for the players to role-play the interaction of the scene together. Fiasco is designed such that all of the players have the same knowledge surrounding the potential paths the story can take, and are afforded the same level of input in determining how to proceed. While dice rolls still impact the story, outcomes are not shaped by the imagination or reaction of a GM, and are instead decided upon by the whole group.

The primary advantage of GM-less games in the context of TA-RPGs is the control it affords players regarding the selection of and approach to content. This freedom encourages players to collaborate and share ideas. Among groups that are willing to speak openly about their goals and encourage each other toward growth, GM-less games can encourage participants to regulate and to challenge each other to engage in scenes that are specifically oriented toward individual and group goals. Such organic and self-directed growth has the potential to rival and overshadow facilitator-directed scenarios and be impactful for all participants involved.

From a TA-RPG perspective, GM-less games present some additional challenges. Without the guidance of a TA-RPG facilitator, it can be difficult for a player to engage in self-directed growth. For example, consider a participant who often backs down from expressing her opinions in conflict and is trying to work on self-advocacy. In a game with a GM, the GM can intentionally create scenarios which provide her scaffolded opportunities to speak up for herself through her character. However, in a GM-less game, this participant may avoid placing her character into situations which allow for scaffolded self-advocacy, or may be placed into situations where her lack of self-advocacy is positively reinforced.

Story Versus Strategy

The goal of all TTRPGs is to tell a story. However, there are two ends of a spectrum for TTRPG game design that approach the method of collaborative storytelling in different ways. On one end is strategy-based TTRPGs, which focus on the direct execution of specific skills, abilities, and actions performed by the characters. On the other end of the spectrum are story-based TTRPGs which focus on wholly narrative-oriented decision-making largely determined directly by the player rather than the specific execution of individual actions performed by a character.

Both strategy- and story-based TTRPGs accomplish the goal of collaboratively telling a story together, but they do so from very different perspectives of player agency and input. In a completely strategy-based TTRPG, the player impacts the environment, and thus the story, completely through the actions and decisions of their character. Games like D&D, Pathfinder, Shadowrun, and 13th Age are all focused largely on strategy-based game design. In these games, the player controls a single character, usually across multiple sessions and storylines. These games focus on specific executable moves of characters (e.g., a thrust attack with a sword, a fire spell that they cast, or a sprinting maneuver). Further, these games often have specific character actions for social encounters (e.g., lying, uncovering a lie, and determining how well they get along with someone). Each action performed by the character has a predefined rule and a specific determination for success, and sometimes additional rules to delineate the outcome of that success. As players continue to experience success and failure through their actions, their characters impact and progress the storyline. Indeed, players have access to a near limitless number of options and are afforded significant agency through their characters' actions.

In a story-based TTRPG, the player may or may not control a singular character. Many story-based games have players controlling several characters at a time, or changing the character that they control depending on the current scene or encounter of the story. Story-based TTRGPs may have players decide character actions, but they focus on having the players impact the narrative of the shared story directly through verbal input, rather than through specific actions that their characters take. In the game Microscope, a GM-less and diceless (see later) game focused on building out a timeline of events, players work together to create a series of interesting events across a vast length of time (i.e., the life of the universe). The game has no GM and does not involve rolling dice. The players make decisions about the kinds of events that take place throughout the timeline, through the placement of cards and discussions regarding what they would like the timeline to contain. They may enact scenes between characters within that timeline, but the outcome of those scenes is determined in a discussion between the players before the scene is started, rather than through dice rolls or character actions that take place during the scene. In this way, though the players may play out a conflict between two characters, both players already know, and are in agreement about, who will win the conflict before it ever begins.

Story-based games are appropriate for groups desiring to create a truly collaborative storytelling experience where all players involved, including the facilitator, are given an equal amount of power to impact the story being told. Similar to GM-less games, discussed earlier in this chapter, story-based games give the players a greater sense of control of and insight into the narrative being told. As a result, they remove an element of mystery from the storyline that the facilitator may incorporate into other types of games.

Story-based games contain several challenges when it comes to building a strong player-to-character relationship. Players who are more involved in the overall story design may see their characters as completely displaced from themselves, disregarding the therapeutic impact of aesthetic distance (discussed in Chapter 5). As a result, players see the character as just a character in a story, and are less likely to be personally impacted by the successes or struggles of the character. When the character grows, the player is less likely to internalize that growth, and thus less likely to experience their own personal growth through it. In such games, TA-RPG facilitators need to focus on the messaging of the story as a whole, and the reflection of the experiences of the players at the table (e.g., how well they collaborate, resolve differences in their visions for the story, or share their thoughts on the story decisions that were made), rather than through the vicarious experiences of the characters.

A lack of strategic decision-making on the part of the player can sometimes cause a purely story-based game to feel repetitive and unending. Strategy-based TTRPGs offer opportunities for the players to overcome in-game obstacles through their character's actions, as well as achieve in-game goals for their character (e.g., unlocking new abilities). Conversely, in story-based games, the only goal in the game is the continued telling of a story together, which is forever the same throughout the life of the game. The lack of variation, and the potential ease in which players can simply craft the story around them, can make story-based games well suited for a single play session. However, play over several weeks, or even years, can feel stagnant and uninteresting.

The incorporation of story-based and strategy-based elements in game design is on a wide spectrum, and many games use both aspects in order to benefit from the advantages that they bring. For instance, in the game

Dungeon World, players control single characters which are played consistently over the course of many sessions. Overall, Dungeon World would appear to leverage a largely strategy-based game design. However, at times the game provides opportunities for players to decide a direction of narrative, rather than to leave that decision to the specific actions of a character. These story-based opportunities in Dungeon World often come in the form of questions that the players can ask the facilitator, which presuppose aspects of the answer. In the basic rules of Dungeon World, the players have a move which can allow them to ask questions such as "What here is useful or valuable to me?" or "What here is not what it appears to be?" Both questions require the facilitator to potentially change the plot and story direction to include something that is useful or valuable, or to be different from how it appears, even if those things were not true to begin with.

From the perspective of TA-RPG facilitation, games which are more focused on a strategy-based rule set are likely to be more useful over the life of a long-lasting group due to providing a consistent opportunity to build personal connection to a single character. Such a process allows character growth to better reflect personal growth for many players. Alternatively, story-based games are usually appropriate for single session play, and for players who are interested and ready for a more fully collaborative story experience where each of the participants can be openly reflective of the way in which the play experience or story is meaningful to them.

Dice-Based and Diceless Systems

One consistent aspect to TTRPGs is the introduction of a randomization tool to help determine the outcome of decisions or actions attempted by, or happening to, the characters in the game. In the context of TTRPGs, this determination of outcomes is sometimes referred to as "conflict resolution." Despite the name, this process does not always represent conflict between characters, but between environmental or story elements that exist in the game. Most commonly, this conflict resolution occurs using a variety of differently shaped dice, often modifying the roll with a bonus or penalty based on character attributes that represent the character's skills and abilities.

A detailed description of the function of a randomization tool is covered in more detail in Chapter 2. The kind of dice or the types of randomizing agents vary significantly across different TTRPGs. D&D's popularity, and its use of seven specific dice, has created a standard to which other game systems are compared. Other game systems, such as the Cortex system, opt to use a larger number of the same kind of dice. For example, resolving conflict by rolling multiple ten-sided dice, with the success determined by the adding up the number of dice that roll over a certain target value.

Dice serve several other functions beyond conflict resolution. Notably, dice provide immediate, tangible feedback that a player's success is, at least partially, dictated by external forces. When a player's actions are unsuccessful, it is easier for that failure to be discarded as a simple result of dice, rather than a poor choice or a personal character flaw. This randomness also provides a jolt of excitement when a roll goes well, especially if the roll is difficult to achieve (i.e., an action requiring a very high dice roll). This can lead to tense and exciting moments within the game and the narrative.

Utilizing dice within one's game also provides opportunities to experience the satisfying tactile sensation of rolling them. Although dice can be rolled electronically through a number of applications, the tactile experience is notably lost in translation. Rolling physical dice is a great way to help players feel engaged in the game, and can spark further interest in the hobby of TTRPGs. Dice come in a broad variety of colors, patterns, textures, and materials, with many players deriving meaning from the acquisition and utilization of their dice as an exercise of personal expression for themselves and their character.

Some TTRPGs do not use dice as a way to create randomization. Commonly, these systems use decks of cards, coins, or other easy ways to generate a random number. A notable example comes from Dread, a horror-based game that uses a stack of blocks, similar to Jenga, to create a rising feeling of potential failure corresponding with the inevitable collapse of the tower. These alternative methods can be captivating to some players, especially if they are used to dice-based games.

Complexity

The complexity of a game is a measure of how difficult it is to understand and execute character creation and rules of play. More complex games offer a deeper level of participant problem solving, focusing on how to maximize the effectiveness of their character or teamwork interactions, either through strategic play or through character creation and specialization. This complexity can be appealing as a way for interested and engaged participants to feel rewarded for their cleverness and deep engagement in the game.

A more complex game also means more rules for the GM and players to maintain and track. For example, in the game Dungeon World, a game dedicated to a less complex and more narrative-driven play, the rules description for a character pushing an enemy backward as a part of their attack is two sentences long and only requires that the player include the push along with their description.

This is in contrast to a game such as Pathfinder (2nd edition), a game known for its complex character building and player character modifiers. In the aforementioned example, a character pushing an enemy backwards as a part of their attack, a player character in Pathfinder cannot even perform the same such an action without having first gained the feat "Bull Rush" within the character creation or leveling process. The bull rush description is over a dozen sentences and three paragraphs long, and details many explicit circumstances and dice rolls which must take place in order to successfully push the enemy. It goes on to describe exactly what the results of such an action would be, and how that may impact the enemy in various circumstances, such as if they get pushed into another enemy. The difference between the two systems is significant in the number and complexity of rules involved to execute the same action.

At first glance, it may seem that a more complex game is not worth the effort to use in a therapeutic context. While a more complex system may seem unwieldy or difficult to learn, it also provides the opportunity for a sense of mastery and the joy of solving a different set of problems. A feeling of mastery can only be accomplished in the face of challenge or difficult obstacles. More complicated rules and conditions for success create additional opportunities for players to feel accomplished in their problem-solving skills and to build a sense of confidence to go along with that accomplishment.

Consider the following metaphor regarding the value of complexity within TA-RPGs. Imagine a middle school student who struggles in their math class. When confronted by their parents to ascertain the root of the problem, the student says, "It is just so boring." Upon learning this, the parents speak to the school and arrange to move the student into a more advanced level of math. In response, the student becomes more engaged and subsequently demonstrates improved performance. Despite the material becoming more challenging, it is that complexity that makes the math class more engaging and interesting. The same can be said for the complexity of game systems.

While a less-complex game may provide more flexibility and simplicity for the player and GM, that very simplicity may also be what makes the game less engaging for certain players and facilitators. This lack of engagement may cause some players to have less fun, resulting in less robust growth. A guiding principle in selecting the complexity of a game should always be informed by the engagement and fun that the participants and facilitator will have. An enthusiastic facilitator who loves a more complex game may be able to engage players who would normally not enjoy something as complex. Similarly, enthusiastic and excited participants will make a more challenging and complicated game more enjoyable through the enthusiasm they bring. In contrast, it is encouraged that a simpler game may be more appropriate for younger participants and those who are new to TTRPGs.

When selecting a game system, D&D holds a number of positive aspects that make it the optimal choice among many facilitators. Its complexity is varied, allowing for rules that are simple to play and learn, alongside multiple optional systems to layer on top of the basic rules for added complexity. Dungeons & Dragons, 5th edition, has streamlined game mechanics with clear directions to players for how to build and play their characters. It provides a wealth of support materials for GMs, including adventure modules, blogs, video materials, and dedicated online repositories for everything from rules adjustments to magic items and custom spells. These support materials can allow less experienced GMs and players to learn the game more easily, as well as answer questions that may come up through the course of play.

In general, game system complexity is an area where the facilitator's mastery of the game is of the utmost importance. A facilitator should avoid using a complex TTRPG system if they constantly feel unsure of the system and struggle to stay organized in the face of complex rules. TA-RPG facilitators will be unable to leverage the full potential of their selected tool (i.e., the game system) if the associated complexity falls outside their range of competence.

Player Age Appropriateness

An important consideration within game selection for TA-RPGs is participant age. Facilitators must be mindful to appropriately match setting and complexity to the developmental level of participants. A horror-themed game, such as Dread, is likely to be inappropriate for young children. Not only is the horror setting a poor choice for that age group, but Dredd requires significant dexterity when using its block tower-based conflict resolution mechanic. Such a choice would make engagement more challenging for players of a younger age due to their less-developed fine motor skills and patience.

Games like Pathfinder or Starfinder, which utilize comparatively more complicated systems, may be inappropriately challenging for a younger age group. The players may find the content difficult to understand or not worthy of the effort needed to engage in the playful and fun parts of the game.

Although age is an important indicator of developmental capacity, it should not be the only determining factor when considering the appropriateness of a game. Some ten-year-old players may have an interest in more complex game mechanics or in settings that might usually be considered age-inappropriate. Whenever possible, it is important to understand the needs and skills of the players participating in the game, rather than to make broad assumptions about their needs and capacities.

There are many TTRPGs that are well suited for younger players. No Thank You Evil! is a simplified TTRPG system designed to build on young players' imaginations, introducing new mechanics into the game slowly as the players learn more about the game. It is bright and colorful, with a setting that allows for tremendous flexibility. Additionally, No Thank You Evil! has no specifically defined genre, allowing players to select wizards, robots, cats, and astronauts as playable characters.

Selecting an age-appropriate game is not always about trying to find games for kids. Often this can mean having a setting or a level of game complexity that best engages the particular life phase and interests of the players at the table. A group of teens that are exploring personal identity might enjoy Vampire: the Masquerade, even though it leans toward a more mature theme and setting. Conversely, a group of adults in their 30s, who have never played a TTRPG before, might benefit from the simplicity of Critical Core.

Setting and Genre

The setting of a TTRPG game remains an incredibly important aspect of game system selection when it comes to participant engagement. A group of participants who are enthusiastic about 17th-century London, complete with all of the historical aspects of that time period, will be much more excited to play a game with a setting that takes place during that time than a game set in outer space. Additionally, some genres or settings may be unfamiliar to participants, and thus difficult to imagine. Participants who have never been exposed to the Star Wars franchise will struggle to understand the significance of an enemy igniting a lightsaber during a climactic battle. In such a scenario, the facilitator's descriptions, and subsequent engagement from the players, are likely to fall flat or remain uninteresting. Choosing the optimal setting requires an understanding of the most relevant cultural backgrounds and interests of the players at the table, as well as a willingness on the facilitator's part to potentially introduce players to their first experience with a particular story genre.

The setting should not be considered a static and unchangeable aspect of the game. A Starfinder game, which commonly takes place in a science fiction setting, could still allow for travel to a new planet that mimics the themes of high fantasy, with dwarves and magic being predominant in the adventure. A horror-themed game can be combined with modern realism to create a game dedicated to hunting down serial killers, rather than battling against ghosts and other worldly monsters. Existing settings can be creatively adjusted, while new game systems and their associated settings continue to be released, containing novel perspectives on classic genres and ways to adjust them to suit a variety of play experiences.

While it is common for a group to experience an entire campaign within the same setting, the narratives of TTRPGs need not be restricted to a single setting. Many stories may bounce between settings and genres, as well as mix multiple genres simultaneously. For example, a game may be set in space (typical of the science fiction genre), focusing on a high school aboard a space station. Simultaneously, a magical creature (typical of the fantasy genre) is invading the school, resulting in elements of fear and chaos for the plays to overcome (typical of the horror genre). Following the resolution of this storyline, the students may crash land upon a desert planet, shifting into a western-themed genre.

It can often be helpful to select a setting that the facilitator and participants are familiar with. Participants who are fans of the Marvel Cinematic Universe may be significantly more invested in a superhero-themed game, while fans of Star Trek may prefer the theme of space exploration. A player's familiarity with a genre can enhance their ability to visualize narrative descriptions, support their imagination and creativity, and provide a shared language to build upon.

The following examples include several common settings among TTRPGs. TA-RPG facilitators should be mindful of which settings resonate most strongly with themselves and their players. Although not an exhaustive list, these examples are meant to inspire facilitators to create their own worlds, as well as to serve as a guide when choosing game systems or modules within the same genre.

High Fantasy

High fantasy has become popularized through literature, television, and film through stories such as the *Lord of the Rings* and *Game of Thrones*, as well as through video game media such as *The Elder Scrolls*, *The Legend of Zelda*, and *Minecraft*. High fantasy settings often contain bows and arrows, knights in metal armor wielding swords and shields, and fantastical races and creatures (e.g., dwarves, elves, and dragons). Additionally, high fantasy commonly contains some form of magic that may present differently from story to story. Typically, this magic, or similar mysterious force, can be manipulated by select individuals and defies the laws of physics and thermodynamics of the real world. This magic often catalyzes important quests, provides a vector for obtaining greater power, and conveniently creates spaces for creative, if not typically impossible, scenarios for players to explore. Popular game systems that utilize the high fantasy setting include the Forgotten Realms campaign setting for Dungeons & Dragons, Pathfinder, 13th Age, and Dungeon World.

Science Fiction

Science fiction centers around not-yet-existing technology and often focuses on interstellar themes. Players are often drawn to the mystique of spaceships, exploration, extraterrestrial species, and alien technology. Similar to magic within the high fantasy setting, advanced technology can serve as a useful tool for GMs looking for a convenient explanation for any continuity errors or to serve as the catalyst for a narrative arc. Notably, science fiction does not need to take place in the future. Games systems like Tales from the Loop take place during the 1980s, while introducing technological advancements with no real-world corollary in order to explore the premise of "what if" these technologies existed at that time. Popular game systems that utilize the science fiction setting include Starfinder, the Star Trek Role-playing Game, and the Star Wars RPG.

Superhero

Superhero themes often take place in a modern era and are defined by the fantastic abilities of select individuals that set them apart from the average person. The fantastic abilities can be gained through any number of means, including advanced technology, mutations, magic, intense training, and blind luck. This genre has grown in popularity due to the rise of DC and Marvel Comics media. Popular game systems that utilize the superhero setting include Masks and Mutants and Masterminds.

Steampunk

The steampunk setting often combines Victorian-era aesthetics with retro-futuristic technology. Steampunk often contains devices and vehicles which mimic the functionality of modern and even future technological devices, but derived from gear and steam engine parts and aesthetics. The mishmash of Victorian looks and advanced technology creates a unique world feeling often akin to magic. Some steampunk themes (e.g., video phone calls, watches, gears, holograms, submarines) can date back to the writings of Jules Verne or H.P. Lovecraft. Steampunk settings rarely occur by themselves and often incorporate elements of other genres (e.g., high fantasy, science fiction, or horror). Popular game systems that utilize the steampunk setting include Blades in the Dark, Iron Kingdoms, and the Eberron campaign setting for D&D.

Horror

Horror games center around themes that bring up fear and the unknown. Many horror games focus on impossibly powerful monsters or unstoppable creatures that chase or threaten to harm the players. Subgenres of horror can include gothic horror (e.g., vampires and werewolves), paranormal horror (i.e., ghosts and haunted houses), realistic horror (e.g., crime), and psychological horror (e.g., phobias, madness, and paranoia). Popular game systems that utilize the horror setting include Dread, Call of Cthulhu, and Alien: The Role-playing Game.

Romance

The romance genre focuses specifically on the interplay of relationships and how they evolve over time. While a romance setting can refer to sexual or romantic relationships between two characters, it does not have to. The genre encompasses many games which simply focus on building relationships rather than overcoming outside obstacles or battling enemies. This genre continues to gain popularity within the RPG community, with prominent examples being relatively recent releases. Some games, such as Star Crossed, explore forbidden love, while other games, such as Thirsty Sword Lesbians, explore queer stories through a system that emphasizes narrative drama and player safety. Monsterhearts, a high school drama TTRPG where every player character is a teenage version of classic monster, is renowned for its approach to contain innovative approaches to sexuality and LGBTQIA+ issues.

Modern Realism

Modern realism is a diverse genre that covers any setting that takes place in the modern era without the inclusion of implausible elements found in the aforementioned genres. These settings typically portray mundane experiences of everyday life, broadly covering everything from high school student experiences to narratives of elite military operations. Popular game systems that utilize the modern realism setting include Fiasco, MASHED, and Noire World.

Historical Realism

Historical Realism is similar to modern realism, but takes place within a specific era of human history prior to the modern era. These games emphasize historical accuracy during periods of history that are often especially important or interesting to the players and facilitators. Common examples include events surrounding the First and Second World Wars, medieval Europe, and feudal Japan. Similar to modern realism, this setting does not include implausible elements found in other genres, instead focusing on contemporaneous technologies and resources that existed during the specific period of time of the game's setting. Popular game systems that utilize the historical realism setting include The Price of Coal: A Story Game of Labor Rights, Carolina Death Crawl, Night Witches, and Good Society.

Popular Media

Settings based on popular media are prevalent, broad, and diverse. Although not always officially licensed, a remarkable number of television shows, comic books, movies, novels, and video games have an associated TTRPG translation based on its setting. Notable examples include Ghostbusters, Teenage Mutant Ninja Turtles, and My Little Pony. Despite considerable variability to the quality of some examples within this genre, they hold significant value in their ability to invoke the imagination and creativity of fans of a specific media.

Mixed Settings

The setting of the game can provide limitless possibilities for imagination and game engagement. A clever and experienced GM can use the interests and culture of their participants to specifically craft and cater the game to maximize their engagement. Even participants who have never played a TTRPG before may become significantly intrigued when it is described as a version of their favorite show, movie, or era of history. Setting and genre are tools in the skilled facilitator's kit that should not be ignored.

Two common options for mixed settings include hybrid settings and shifting settings. GMs who are interested in facilitating a game with a hybrid setting may seek game systems that intentionally blend two or more genres simultaneously. For example, Monsterhearts blends elements of romance, modern realism, and horror. GMs who are interested in facilitating a game with a shifting setting may seek game systems that specifically focus on moving between genres as a direct function of the game's mechanics. The Strange, a predominantly science fiction game set in a modern age, playfully defies and expands upon its baseline setting by consistently providing players opportunities to move between dimensions in a manner that mimics each of the aforementioned setting options. Additionally, many well-established game systems (e.g., D&D, Pathfinder, and Numenera) may originate from a specific setting, but provide a broad selection of expanded materials with additional setting options and narrative explanations for moving between these various settings. For example, the Planescape campaign setting for D&D narratively links all other potential settings together through a hub of interdimensional magical portals found within Sigil, the "City of Doors." Such contrivances can serve as a convenient setting in and of itself, allowing players centralized crossroads to transition between shifting settings and providing a consistent location to serve as a hybrid setting, welcoming an infinite number of characters and elements from other settings. Similar examples of such locations include Yggdrasil, The World Tree, from Norse mythology, the Wood Between the Worlds described in The Magician's Nephew by C.S. Lewis, and the Neitherlands described in Lev Grossman's The Magicians.

There are also many game systems designed to have no particular defined setting or genre, boasting the ability to be made into any setting that the players and GM desire. These games often have supplemental materials to help GMs focus on a specific genre, while leaving things open-ended enough to allow one to craft their own hybrid setting or shifting setting. Popular game systems that utilize various styles of mixed settings include FATE, GURPS, Shadowrun, and No Thank You Evil!.

Culture and Identity

An important responsibility of every TA-RPG facilitator is the consideration and, when appropriate, incorporation of the cultures and personal histories of the players at the table. As discussed in Chapter 7, having a game experience that incorporates personal cultural history, or responds to the personal lived experiences of the players in regards to their identity or culture, can be affirming and validating. GMs can insert cultural references into the story, the setting's culture and history, or non-player characters (NPCs), but game selection, on its own, can also be a powerful way to build affirming and accepting worlds that help players feel a greater sense of safety and belonging at the table. Coyote and Crow serves as an exemplar of the inclusion of Indigenous populations' culture in a game setting. It is a hybrid science fiction and fantasy game developed by an all native, First Nations identified, team. It is set in a First Nations alternate future where colonization never happened, and provides imagery and storytelling tools to help build on this engaging setting. A game like Coyote and Crow provides an opportunity to build on a cultural perspective that may be especially meaningful for the players at the table. Players who come from this specific cultural background or identity may find the opportunity to play within this setting and ruleset to be affirming, providing further opportunities for insight within their play. Further, players who do not identify with this culture may still find the opportunity to learn more about it to be unique and inviting.

Cultural history is not the only setting design that facilitators should consider based on the personal history or identity of the participating players. Personal identity, such as sexual or gender identity, is also an important consideration that facilitators should consider in the creation or selection of their game and setting. Selecting a game like Monsterhearts, mentioned earlier in this chapter, in order to help create a safe and welcoming TTRPG experience for LGBTQIA+ identified players can help them to feel both affirmed in their safety within the group and more free to express themselves through their character. It is an important job of any therapeutic GM to consider and balance all of these aspects when selecting the game or adjusting the setting and contents of the game world.

Getting Started

This chapter has explored multiple facets of TTRPG design and their potential application for intentional growth in therapeutic settings. However, with so many variables to consider, it may be overwhelming for inexperienced TA-RPG facilitators to select the optimal game for themselves and their group. If in doubt regarding game selection, we recommend TA-RPG facilitators start with TTRPGs that utilize a GM role, a strategy-based design, and a dice-based system. While experienced therapeutic GMs may choose to deviate from these recommendations, such choices should be intentional, be informed by clinical theory, and serve a specific function (e.g., accommodating population considerations or achieving specific outcomes). In addition to being a convenient starting point for inexperienced TA-RPG facilitators, most of the techniques and examples throughout this text refer to these game-design aspects. Though many techniques outlined in other sections of this book apply across TTRPGs, some will necessitate these qualities.

Choose a Game With a Game Master Role

There are numerous advantages to the facilitator serving as the GM. Key among them is the substantial increase in control the facilitator has over the narrative. As the GM, the TA-RPG facilitator is empowered to guide encounters to align with specific areas of growth. Further, this role allows facilitators to filter input from participants that may be inappropriate or antithetical to group goals.

Choose a Strategy-Based Game

Due to their complexity (e.g., leveling mechanics and clearly defined character traits and abilities), strategy-based games are uniquely suited to groups that meet to tell a continuous story over time. Despite increased complexity, many new players express appreciation for the clear order of operations and concise list of actions that are associated with strategy-based games. Players can readily perceive their character's relative strengths and weaknesses, learn through observation of others, and leverage added structure in service of creativity. These qualities instill a strong desire to return sessions after session, encouraging players to consistently move toward personal goals in and out of the game.

Choose a Dice-Based System

Despite the variation in randomizing agents across games, dice hold a special place in the hearts of many players. The appreciation and collection of dice serves as a hobby in and of itself, offering another connection point for shared experiences between players. Their multifaceted designs feature a range of diverse tactile and visual experiences, including coloration, texture, and weight. Due to the prolific use of the six-sided die in other games, players who are new to TTRPGs will often adapt well to understanding how to use dice, and will appreciate their novelty when holding and rolling dice with an unusual number of sides. Further, due to variation in dice shape (i.e., number of sides), individual dice can represent variable success criteria and provide a specific range of potential outcomes.

Choose a Game With Magic in the Setting

There are many settings to choose from, but settings infused with magic (e.g., fantasy settings) allow GMs to satisfactorily explain challenges, solutions, plot holes, and other narrative contrivances of their game. While modern realism settings may be optimal for some groups, magical settings provide a novel experience for those interested in exploring stories and overcoming challenges beyond the real world.

Choose a Game With Available Resources and Supplements

New GMs need not reinvent the wheel, especially in isolation. Selecting a TTPRG with readily available resources can reduce the creative burden of TA-RPG facilitators. Although some TTRPGs present a high financial cost of entry, most feature affordable starter sets or core rulebooks that reduce barriers to participation. Further, some TTRPGs are supported by numerous publications and other resources, providing additional narrative hooks, whole story modules, advanced rules, and expanded universes. Some TTRPGs are also supported by online websites dedicated to digital material and/or communities dedicated to unofficially published compatible material.

Modules

Modules are the outline or guide to be used by a GM to facilitate an adventure. They typically include information about the specific setting, NPCs, possible goals for the party, as well as obstacles the party will encounter. Modules can be detailed and complex or streamlined and simple guidelines for the story the group will tell. Most modules are designed to align with a specific game system though some can be altered to fit other similar systems by experienced GMs. TA-RPG facilitators can create their own modules or use published modules, which can be an amazing resource for TA-RPG groups. If using a published module, the facilitator should read through the module as part of their group preparation, identify areas that can be utilized to support the group goals, and make adjustments to content as needed for appropriateness and group fit. Published modules typically fall in one of two categories:

Official Modules

Many game system designers have designed story modules to go along with their games, and to keep players interested and engaged in their particular game system. Official materials are often created by a team of writers, are given game design oversight for balance, and often have had an extensive review and edit process.

Unofficial Modules

The TTRPG community has contributed many storylines and modules across game systems. Popular games with many players have more options, but even less popular games have online followings creating interesting story and world content and making them available online. Some of these can be purchased from game stores, but a majority of unofficial modules are available in digital formats through websites like drivethruRPG.com and DMs Guild, among others. One danger to these unofficial modules is that they vary significantly in quality, content, and game balance. These materials are not made by the creators of the original game system for which they were designed, and even professional looking materials may have been created by a single person without oversight or accountability. Many of the potential pitfalls of unofficial materials can be mitigated by utilizing well-reviewed modules, well-known third-party publishers, or simply by reading through the material thoroughly before using it in a group.

Many GMs use completely custom- designed game experiences, created by the GM specifically for, and sometimes with, the players at the table (see the section on Collaborative Worldbuilding, Chapter 11). This is colloquially referred to as a "homebrew" campaign or adventure. Homebrew campaigns have many advantages, including the ability to create stories which specifically speak to the needs of each player or character. However, building story and campaign elements from scratch can require significantly more work, planning, and knowledge of TTRPGs settings and rules.

The distinction between published modules and homebrew adventures is somewhat of a false dichotomy. In any well-run TTRPG group, the facilitator will adjust the content to best serve the needs and interests of the group, which means that the same module, run for two different groups, may look wildly different based on participant decisions and facilitator responses.

Regardless of the type of module used, the story outline and module encounters should always be seen as helpful guidelines, never rigid rules. As TA-RPGs are a collaborative storytelling experience, the players, as well as the facilitator, have input into where the story goes next. When utilizing a module of any kind, the facilitator should feel comfortable adjusting the module as needed—whether that means switching around the layout of rooms, adjusting the difficulty of an obstacle, or adjusting the content to be more engaging to the group. Many TTRPG GMs, and TA-RPG facilitators, find modules to be a powerful source of inspiration and feel comfortable adjusting those stories to help maintain a collaborative experience for their players.

Conclusion

TA-RPG facilitators must consider numerous variables when selecting a game system that best suits the needs and interests of their players. Although the preponderance of options may be overwhelming at times, maintaining a focus on popularity, complexity, setting, and culture will serve a facilitator well. Dungeons & Dragons, 5th edition, may be a great place for new GMs to start. Due to its popularity, it is recommended that all TA-RPG facilitators be at least passingly familiar with it, and while many TTRPGs contain the qualities found in this chapter, none have the name recognition of D&D. Ultimately, TA-RPG facilitators must strike a balance between selecting a game system in which they are competent and familiar, and one that directly and auspiciously supports participants' growth.

Critical Core, a TTRPG created and distributed by Game to Grow, was designed specifically with the qualities outlined in this chapter, providing guidance and tools to help new facilitators get started using TTRPGs as a therapeutic tool. Critical Core features a streamlined and easy to learn set of rules specifically designed for new players and new GMs, complete with a facilitator's guide that applies the approaches of this text, modules focused on specific areas of growth for neurodiverse youth, and a setting that works well for participants ranging in age from ten to adulthood. Physical copies of Critical Core include dice, a GM screen, a dry erase gridded play mat, and spell and ability cards to help players understand their character's available actions. Most importantly, Critical Core is compatible with all tools, suggestions, and therapeutic techniques contained in this text, integrating the very approaches and philosophies of the Game to Grow Method into its design. More information about Critical Core can be found at criticalcore.org.

Regardless of selection, no game will ever perfectly fit all members of a group, and therapeutic GMs should be ready and able to shift to another game system or adjust both the game world and the play experiences to best serve the players at the table.

Games Referenced in This Chapter

13th Age
Alien: The Role-playing Game
Blades in the Dark
Call of Cthulhu
Carolina Death Crawl
Cortex System
Coyote and Crow
Critical Core
Dungeons and Dragons
Dungeon World
Dread
Eberron campaign setting for D&D
FATE
Fiasco
Ghostbusters
Good Society
GURPS
Iron Kingdoms
MASHED
Masks
Microscope
Monsterhearts
Mutants and Masterminds
My Little Pony
Night Witches
Noire World
No Thank You Evil
Pathfinder
Shadowrun
Star Crossed
Starfinder
Tales from the Loop
Teenage Mutant Ninja Turtles
The Price Of Coal: A Story Game of Labor Rights

The Star Trek Role-playing Game
The Star Wars RPG
The Strange
Thirsty Sword Lesbians
Vampire: The Masquerade

Reference

Roll20. (2022, February 28). The Orr Group industry report Q4 2021. *Roll20 Blog*. Retrieved July 25, 2022, from https://blog.roll20.net/posts/the-orr-report-q4-2021/

7

Population Considerations in Therapeutically Applied Role-Playing Games

As discussed in Chapter 5, the Game to Grow Method of TA-RPGs is a relational model, where the impetus for change is grounded in the relationships built through play and process. To this end, facilitators need to create an accessible and safe environment for their participants to effectively build such relationships. Though this chapter specifically includes sections about diversity, accessibility, and inclusion, we encourage readers to note the ways in which these topics are woven throughout the rest of the book. Effective inclusion practices and cultural competency is an integral part of the Game to Grow Method of TA-RPGs and should not be considered adjunctive. In this chapter, we will discuss accessibility in TA-RPGs, diversity, and inclusion through the lens of cultural humility, the history of discrimination within tabletop role-playing games (TTRPGs), and recommendations when working with selected clinical populations.

Accessibility

There are currently a multitude of tools available to increase the accessibility of TTRPGs (Kretchmer, 2020; Sjunneson, 2019). Though continued progress in accessibility is needed in the TTRPG space, facilitators should feel comfortable identifying and making accommodations available to their participants as needed. When identifying appropriate accommodations, the goal for increasing accessibility is to increase an individual's access to the game and group while maintaining the autonomy of the participant.

For example, regarding a participant who is unable to manipulate small objects, such as physical dice, potential accommodations include rolling dice for the participant, providing the participant large format dice that are easier to grasp and roll, or providing the participant with a voice- or touch-activated digital dice roller. Assuming the participant is able to use all three of these accommodations, the first accommodation (rolling dice for them) removes the most autonomy over the

DOI: 10.4324/9781003281962-7

participant's dice rolling, while the second and third accommodations keep the agency of rolling dice with the participant.

Participants should be included in the decision-making process about which accommodations to use. When working with a participant to select the most appropriate accommodations, the facilitator should be aware of the roadblocks to inclusion many individuals with disabilities face. Individuals with disabilities have experienced barriers to accommodations including stigma, procedural issues, and lack of instructor support for accommodations (Quinlan et al., 2012). Additionally, students with disabilities commonly downplay their disability status when seeking accommodations (Barnard-Brak et al., 2010; Magnus & Tøssebro, 2012). Because of stigma and challenges accessing accommodations, participants may be more likely to use the accommodation that is the least disruptive for others, as opposed to the accommodation that best fits their goals and preferences for the group. Depending on the setting and relationship with the participant, it may be appropriate to preface the list of potential accommodations with your goals for the participant's inclusion and participation, as well as an explicit message that use of any accommodations is normal, valid, and accepted within the group.

Commonly Used Accommodations in TTRPGs

- Braille dice
- Screen readers
- Large print dice/fonts
- Closed captioning services
- Chat functions
- Dyslexic-friendly character sheets
- Fidget devices
- Shared session notes

Diversity and Inclusion

Cultural Humility

When developing a TA-RPG group, it is important to consider the communities and individual identities of the group members, as well as the ways in which those identities intersect and inform each member's experience in the world. We encourage facilitators to utilize an approach centered around cultural humility, a process commonly applied to research, mental health care, and physical health care. Cultural humility is a practice of self-reflection, learning, perspective taking, and collaboration to create more genuine, effective, and egalitarian relationships between individuals (Yeager & Bauer-Wu, 2013). In the context of TA-RPGs, similar to any clinical practice, the process of cultural humility is intended to support facilitators approaching their participants from a place of "informed not knowing" (Keenan, 2004). The facilitator should take intentional steps to become informed about common experiences, beliefs, language, and culture of a community, as well as to understand that such learning does not replace or supersede the lived experience of those in the community. Additionally, facilitators should be up-to-date on applicable research that explores the ways in which culture can inform clinical practice (Yeager & Bauer-Wu, 2013). The process of cultural humility is distinct from cultural competence, as an emphasis on achieving "competence" can lead to an approach in which the clinician is falsely perceived as the expert on the client's experience (Sadusky & Yarhouse, 2020).

When using TA-RPGs with any population, the facilitator should adapt participation structure, narrative, and mechanics to fit within community norms and beliefs. For example, if working within a population whose religious beliefs preclude the use of magic (including fictional use depicted in games), a facilitator may utilize a TTRPG system that does not include or rely on magic or magic users. Additionally, though the onus of facilitator education should be on the facilitator, not the participants, the facilitator should continually seek feedback from multiple sources regarding fit and feel of the mechanics and story.

Identities of Players and Characters

Every participant in a TA-RPG group is multifaceted, holding multiple intersecting identities. When considering identities, it is important to understand that parts of an individual's identity (e.g., race, sexual orientation, or religious affiliation) do not exist within a vacuum, but are influenced by each other. For example, a Black woman's experience of sexism in the United States is often different from a White woman's experience of sexism in the United States (McMahon & Kahn, 2016).

Models such as the ADDRESSING framework encourage facilitators to consider multiple aspects of diversity including age, developmental and acquired disabilities, religion, ethnicity, socioeconomic status, sexual orientation, Indigenous heritage, national origin, and gender (Hays, 2008). Though these frameworks are not exhaustive, they can create a foundation from which to explore other salient aspects of identity, including military veteran status, occupation, and parental status. In addition to considering the known or assumed identities of group participants, facilitators should spend time reflecting on how their own identity and lived experiences may influence the group, game, and mechanics. It is important for facilitators to consider the areas in which they hold privilege, especially when other group members are assumed to not hold such privileges. Additionally, facilitators should seek to be aware of where their own identities may be assumed, and make intentional, client-focused decisions regarding disclosure (Hanson, 2005; Knox & Hill, 2003). Invisible and easily concealed identities, such as sexual orientation, disability status, and religious orientation, may be commonly assumed by participants.

Many TTRPGs have mechanics associated with character identities, such as a character's profession, background, and race or species. These mechanics are typically intended to influence game play by outlining rules to support the narrative experience. For example, a character with a sailor background may have the knowledge and skill needed to sail a ship, while a character who used to be a librarian may have an easier time engaging in research or finding a book in a library compared to their teammates. Historically, many TTRPGs have had mechanics tied not only to a character's profession and background but also to their race or species (Garcia, 2017). In part because of the established history of racist portrayals of real-world races through problematic fantasy tropes, some TTRPG systems are moving away from race-based mechanics (Garcia, 2017; Wizards RPG Team, 2020). Racial mechanics can make visible the implicit advantages or disadvantages of certain identities that are reflected in the real world. Even if explicit conversation about identity is unlikely to come up in a game, facilitators should be aware of the ways in which assigning point values to aspects of identity may impact a player's experience of the game and the group. For example, racial bonuses to specific abilities can prioritize the selection of one character race over another, leading players to choose a race less aligned with their preferences or start the game at a disadvantage.

Character Customization

Many TA-RPG groups will use premade character sheets. Such a choice can streamline the character creation process for groups and be especially helpful for individuals who are new to TTRPGs, as well as for groups within settings that may necessitate a rolling roster of participants (e.g., short stay units within hospitals). Whether characters are built from scratch or premade, options for customizing the character to better suit the participant and align with the participant's identities should be clearly available. This customization may include aspects such as physical appearance, background, culture, and disability. There are multiple resources available to support representation of disability and accommodations (i.e., wheelchairs, service animals, canes; Thompson, 2020; Sjunneson, 2019).

Story and World Recommendations

Facilitators should be mindful of the ways in which their game reflects real life. Players may assume that the world presented within the game is the way the game master (GM) thinks the world *should* be. For example, settings that replicate the patriarchal, colonialist governance structure of many western nations may errantly communicate that such a structure is "correct," "preferred," or "universally appropriate."

When considering the inclusion of discrimination within the game's narrative, it is important to be aware of one's own privilege and assumed privilege, as well as the goals and preferences of the group members. Participants may want to adventure in a world in which discrimination exists (either directed at them or others), especially when players and their characters are empowered to positively shift such dynamics. TA-RPGs can be a great opportunity for players to feel empowered and make meaningful change within the collective narrative. However, not all participants will find the replication of discriminatory behaviors or systems empowering. It is also important to note that experiencing discrimination as an individual, as well as observing discrimination directed toward others with a shared identity, can contribute to negative mental health outcomes (Ozier et al., 2019; Mays & Cochran, 2001; Sellers et al., 2006; Yip et al., 2008; Hackett et al., 2019; Ríos-Salas & Larson, 2015). Though more research in this area is needed to better understand where in-game replication is helpful versus harmful, anecdotal reports provide some clues to answering this question. First, participant preference should be prioritized. Participants may not want to navigate simulated discrimination that replicates the genuine discrimination they experience in their daily life, even if they have more power to change problematic systems in the fantasy space. Additionally, the relevance to participant and group goals should be considered. Even if portrayal of discrimination in game is related to participant goals (such as self-advocacy), representation of discrimination in game is likely not the only way to support such goals. Discrimination-related content is likely to increase the psychological stress of an in-game encounter. If participants are already at their capacity for successful regulation, adding an emotionally valent, hurtful experience is likely to push participants into a state of dysregulation, a state inconsistent with efficient learning. Additionally, it may be particularly problematic to portray discriminatory themes when the facilitator holds identities that are similar to the regular perpetrators of discrimination within the lives of the participants. Playing a character, as a GM or player, never gives an individual free reign to engage in harmful or discriminatory behavior.

Facilitators should listen to voices and perspectives beyond their own. They should consume media and participate in games created and run by individuals with experiences and backgrounds different from theirs. Requests made by participants about the people, places, and systems they want to see in the narrative world should be respected. Additionally, facilitators should be mindful that depictions of concepts such as race, gender, and disability are not defined by the game developer or GM alone. These concepts are expanded upon by the group through the collaborative process of group storytelling and experience within TTRPGs (Garcia, 2017).

Customization for Unique Settings

Many TTRPG systems are based in high-fantasy settings, which often resemble a fantasy medieval Europe (Dhar, 2020). Even if high-fantasy settings are the preferred backdrop for the group's stories, they do not have to resemble the political or societal structures common with these settings. For example, the societies may be largely matriarchal, or the countries have a democratic and egalitarian political structure. Facilitators and their participants are encouraged to dream big and to consider The Enthusiasm Doctrine when presenting their game's setting. As discussed in Chapter 11, The Enthusiasm Doctrine encourages GMs to "bend or break whatever rules [they] want . . . to encourage vivacious whole brained engagement in authentic relational play." Thinking *beyond* the way settings are typically portrayed can stretch participants' imagination and help them adapt to a constantly changing world (McGonigal, 2022).

Supporting Participant Responses to Topics of Accessibility, Diversity, and Inclusion

At times, participants in TA-RPG groups may have competing knowledge or sensitivity related to discrimination and language (e.g., racism and/or sexism). This can lead to players using inappropriate language, as well as disagreement around what topics or themes to include in the group. It is the facilitator's responsibility to create opportunities for learning and growth while supporting the safety of the whole group. Further, the growth and learning of one player should not supersede the safety of any other group members. Prior to the start of any group, the facilitator should set expectations about safety and inclusivity through conversations with participants, as well as through the language found on the facilitator's website or paperwork.

Setting behavioral expectations and group norms, such as through using no/please lists (discussed in Chapter 13), increases the likelihood for a successful group. However, this is not a failsafe strategy. There may be times when participants challenge game content or engage in discriminatory behaviors (e.g., microaggressions or slurs) toward other participants, player characters, or non-player characters (NPCs). Supporting adaptive dialogues between participants about sensitive topics is encouraged (Bemak & Chung, 2018). Facilitators may benefit from considering likely topics that may come up within their games and plan possible ways to respond. This preparation can increase the facilitator's comfort level and ability to respond in the moment.

A Tale From the Real-World Table

During an established TA-RPG group with young adolescents, one of the participants, Cole, became frustrated with the actions of another player, and used an ableist slur when expressing his frustration. The players around the table froze, shock clear on their faces. In response, Cole's expression shifted from one of frustration and anger to uncertainty and confusion. The facilitator considered Cole's rapid change in demeanor when viewing the rest of the player's shock, and hypothesized that Cole may not have understood the impact of their words. With a gentle and calm tone, the facilitator said, "Hey Cole, I can see you were pretty upset and were trying to express your feelings when you used that word. That word has been used to really hurt groups of people in the past, so we don't use it anymore. From your current facial expression, I'm guessing you might not have known that part—am I correctly understanding what happened?" Cole expressed that they had not understood the intense impact the word would have—voicing that they did not think it would be a "big deal." The rest of the players visibly relaxed. One of the other players spoke up and stated they also did not know about the impact of the slur until recently. The facilitator's use of functional analysis and assuming best possible intent consistent with the facts helped them to not escalate the situation further, and created opportunities for learning and safety among the group members.

History of TTRPGs and Discrimination

The collaborative and flexible nature of TTRPGs can create a powerful context to foster inclusion and community. However, TTRPG spaces have not and are not always inclusive and welcoming spaces. Historically, many of the developers of TTRPGs have been White, cis, and male, with their viewpoints and biases being heavily emphasized in the TTRPG community (Dhar, 2020; Peterson, 2012; Witwer, 2016). Additionally, high-fantasy and horror genres, which have influenced the development of TTRPG systems and stories, include seminal and prolific writers whose personal character and narrative content have been critiqued for sexist, racist, and ableist content and themes (Fimi, 2022; Blackmoore et al., 2019).

An ongoing conversation in art and gaming spheres focus on whether it is possible or wise to separate art from artist, with the acknowledgment that an artist's beliefs and biases are often implicitly (or explicitly) present in their work. Similarly, TTRPGs are created by people, and their biases are embedded within the systems they create (Garcia, 2017). For TA-RPG facilitators, a basic understanding of the current and historical inclusion challenges of the TTRPG space is necessary to create safe and inclusive gaming spaces.

Modern TTRPGs first emerged in the 1970s, with the 1st edition of Dungeons & Dragons, created by Dave Arneson and Gary Gygax (1974). Early editions of the game used only male pronouns for players and GMs, even after referencing women players (Gygax, 1978). Notably, should players choose to play a female character, her strength score in this fantasy role-playing game (RPG) was capped lower than a male character's potential (Garcia, 2017).

Additionally, a character's race has historically determined skills, abilities, and personality characteristics above and beyond that character's background and origin story (Garcia, 2017). Though more conversation and subsequent changes to mechanics and lore have happened in the TTRPG community in the last decade, an awareness of systems' origins and flaws is important to create an inclusive table. Garcia (2017) outlines the changes in representation of sex and race throughout the subsequent versions of Dungeons & Dragons (D&D) and Pathfinder (1st edition).

J.R.R. Tolkien is often cited as the "father" of modern high-fantasy literature. Some of his stories and descriptions, especially those of orcs and elves have sparked fierce debates among the fantasy and gaming communities regarding the presence (or lack thereof) of racist allegories and underpinnings (Fimi, 2022). The influences of H.P. Lovecraft and his creation, Cthulhu, permeate the horror genre of "Weird fiction." Much of his writing includes overtly racist metaphors and imagery, and evidence of his racist views exists in multiple instances of personal correspondence (Romano, 2020). Inspiration from these literary giants has been carried forward into fantasy writing and TTRPG alike, often without the intention of perpetuating discriminatory ideas or imagery.

Some TTRPG designers explicitly acknowledge this problematic lineage in their materials, such as the reflection found in *Fate of Cthulhu*, developed by Evil Hat Productions. In the manual, the authors acknowledge H.P. Lovecraft, whose work inspired *Fate of Cthulhu*, as racist and antisemitic (Blackmoore et al., 2019). Additionally, many developers have adjusted what is canon to reflect more inclusive, anti-racist ideals, such as the optional changes to racial abilities and alignments introduced by Wizards of the Coast in *Tasha's Cauldron of Everything* (Wizards RPG Team, 2020).

In recent years, increased diversity among game developers has led to system and setting options that sidestep many of the concerns related to historical content, bringing much-needed diversity to the TTG world. These include settings like the Wagadu Chronicles, an African-inspired

Dungeons & Dragons 5e setting developed by Twin Drums, as well as TTRPG systems like Coyote and Crow, which is set in an alternate future where colonization never occurred.

Though progress has been made within TTRPGs and the broader gaming community, discrimination and inclusion concerns related to race, gender, disability, and other identities remain common.

Clinical Populations

TA-RPGs are appropriate for use with a wide variety of diagnoses and experiences. To illustrate this, the authors have chosen to highlight a few diagnoses to discuss common goals, experiences, and recommendations. As with any diagnosis or identity, the goals and recommendations reflected in the following are not applicable to every person with the diagnosis or experience.

Autism Spectrum Disorder

Diagnostically, autism spectrum disorder (ASD) is a form of neurodivergence and is identified through impairments in language and communication, challenges with reciprocal social interaction, and engagement in restricted and repetitive behaviors (APA, 2022; WHO, 2019). Individuals exhibiting the aforementioned challenges may experience functional consequences throughout their lives. Learning, especially in the context of social environments, may be negatively impacted by deficits in social and communication abilities. Further, adaptive skills (e.g., eating, sleeping, and physical hygiene), routine care (e.g., medical appointments and haircuts), academic achievement, and establishing independence may be stifled by strict adherence to routine and aversion to change (APA, 2022; WHO, 2019). Alongside these challenges, individuals with ASD also contend with stigma surrounding their diagnosis. Stigma related to ASD can result in autistic youth being more susceptible to rejection and loneliness compared to neurotypical peers (Kinnear et al., 2015; Bauminger & Kasari, 2000; Bauminger et al., 2003). Autistic individuals are more likely than their neurotypical peers to experience peer victimization and bullying (Maïano et al., 2016). Additionally, research has found that autistic adults may experience heightened feelings of perceived burden to others, thwarted belonging (e.g., insufficient reciprocal relationships), and trauma than non-autistic adults (Pelton et al., 2020). A notable contributing factor influencing ASD stigma appears to be found in the "double-empathy problem" (Milton, 2012). This theory posits that people will struggle to empathize with one another when there are significant discrepancies in their experiences of the world (e.g., first languages, age, executive functioning). Concepts like the "double-empathy problem" highlight the challenges society has with respecting and adapting to individuals with non-normative interaction styles (Milton, 2012). In order to make friends and fit in with peer groups and adults, many autistic individuals compensate for this discrepancy by masking their symptoms or behaviors to appear more normative (Cook et al., 2018; Hull et al., 2021; Pearson & Rose, 2021). However, misguided interventions that train autistic individuals to present as closely to their neurotypical peers as possible can be traumatizing to the individual and may lead to negative long term mental health outcomes (Shkedy et al., 2020; Miller et al., 2021).

Common goals for autistic individuals in TA-RPG groups include finding others to participate in hobbies/shared interests, accessing opportunities for positive social interaction, building interpersonal skills such as meta-communication, and finding social acceptance. A study of autistic youth in Japan found engaging in TTRPGs supported interpersonal communication skills and self-reported quality of life (Kato, 2019). TA-RPG groups should be a social setting in which individuals will not be rejected for often-stigmatized behaviors or experiences, such as repetitive movements or noises, or sensory sensitivities.

TTRPGs can support the use of meta-communication, a secondary communication about how the initial communication should be interpreted. Meta-communication includes the act of communicating about communication and can occur before, during, or after a particular interaction. Meta-communication in play is often used to coordinate roles and plan game play (de Haan et al., 2021). This occurs in TTRPGs whenever players discuss what their characters are planning to do, or how they think and feel. Holding the role of both player and character allows participants to speak for their character, and provide follow-up context or information to interpret the character's actions—similar to the utility of a narrator in a book, play, or movie. Some autistic individuals struggle with the meta-communication skills needed to shift between the in-game world and the out-of-game world (Douglas & Stirling, 2012). TA-RPGs can be a safe space for autistic individuals to gain experience interacting with a complex social world through the game. This game space can allow for increased reflection and decision-making, reduced stakes for misunderstandings, and opportunities for immediate reinforcement of practice of challenging skills. For example, a participant who is not yet interested in making friends with other participants due to past social trauma may have the opportunity to explore the costs and benefits of friendship through an NPC played by the facilitator. The facilitator can provide reinforcement of the participant's efforts for relationship building through the reactions of the NPC, scaffolding the participant's skills as needed. Over time, the participant may gain confidence in their interpersonal skills, resulting in increased feelings of safety with the facilitator and the group as a whole. The facilitator could then provide opportunities for the participant to develop friendships with the other participants. It is important that the participant drives the facilitator's next steps, that is, that the participant is not explicitly directed to make friends with the other participants or NPCs.

Attention Deficit Hyperactivity Disorder

Attention deficit hyperactivity disorder (ADHD) is characterized by difficulties in executive functioning, including challenges with regulating attention and mood, planning, task initiation, perspective taking, and impulsivity (APA, 2022; WHO, 2019). Individuals with ADHD often experience impairments that impact their performance in education, work, and social contexts (APA, 2022; WHO, 2019). Common treatment for ADHD includes stimulant medication and behavioral interventions (Caye et al., 2019). Behavioral interventions can include training for parents, direct intervention with the individual, and accommodations in work and school environments.

Like autism, individuals with ADHD are neurodivergent. Individuals with ADHD can often face stigma related to their challenges, as well as frequent misunderstandings in relationships with peers and family members. Such experiences can negatively impact life satisfaction, mental well-being, and treatment engagement for individuals with ADHD (Mueller et al., 2012). Research exploring ADHD stigma found that many people believe ADHD symptoms are socially inappropriate and childish, and that the presentation of common ADHD behaviors can increase the likelihood of hostility from and rejection by peers (Canu & Carlson, 2003; Stroes et al., 2003; Paulson et al., 2005). Common goals for individuals with ADHD in TA-RPGs include engagement in positive social interactions, increased insight, decreased impulsivity, and enhanced ability to plan.

TA-RPGs can be a validating and supportive environment to improve confidence and well-being by developing skills and highlighting an individual's strengths. The low-risk nature and fantastical settings of TA-RPGs create opportunities for participants to be celebrated for behaviors that may not be adaptive in many other areas of their life. For example, a participant's willingness to act quickly (what in other contexts would be "impulsive behavior") may be exactly what is needed when a local wizard's magic goes awry and the heroes need to rush into a burning library to save them. Additionally, the use of an avatar affords participants valuable aesthetic distance (Chapter 5) between themselves and their character from which to view both their characters and their own struggles and failures. Such insight can support the player's regulation skills, their ability to reflect upon their own behavior, and to problem-solve future challenges. The use of meta-communication in game, as well as reflections from players and the facilitator, can create opportunities to discuss how a character's actions worked (or did not) in a supportive manner for the participant.

Post-traumatic Stress Disorder/History of Trauma

Individuals with a diagnosis of post-traumatic stress disorder (PTSD) have experienced a traumatic event, and continue to experience disruptions to their regulatory system and thought patterns more than a month after the event (APA, 2022; WHO, 2019). The diagnostic criteria for PTSD includes symptoms such as intrusive memories, avoidance of internal and external reminders of the event, maladaptive changes in thinking related to self, others, and the world, as well as disruptions in mood, sleep, and emotional regulation. Individuals with a history of trauma may experience challenges developing appropriate trust with themselves and others, engaging in appropriate risk taking, and participating in valued hobbies and work.

Many of the effective treatments for trauma include intentional and regulated exposure to currently avoided stimuli that are negatively impacting the client's life (Foa et al., 2007; Resick et al., 2016; Shapiro, 2017). For example, treatment for a client who was bitten by a dog may include looking at pictures of dogs, sitting in a room across from a dog, and/or petting a friendly dog, typically in a gradual, sequential manner. In some treatment approaches, the client may be asked to repeatedly recount the story of the trauma while being supported and monitored by a trained clinician to decrease the amount of arousal the client experiences in reaction to the memory (Foa et al., 2007; Shapiro, 2017).

TA-RPGs can be utilized, with the consent of participants, by facilitators trained to do such work to support re-engagement with currently avoided, yet valued activities (e.g., petting a dog). At this time, there is no research to support the replication of traumatic events within TA-RPGs (e.g., the party members experiencing a dog attack). In keeping with the recommendations for group treatments for trauma, such as Cognitive Processing Therapy, facilitators should not intentionally replicate trauma content in TA-RPG groups (Resick et al., 2016). In trauma-focused treatment groups, participants are typically encouraged to talk about the ways in which their trauma impacts their daily lives and share stories of recovery, without sharing specific details leading up to or occurring during the event (Resick et al., 2016). These boundaries support other participants who may be triggered by such details, as well as reduce the potential for comparing each other's traumas. This expectation should be made clear to participants at the beginning of the group, and safety tools should be identified and agreed upon by the group should a participant or facilitator unintentionally introduce content replicating a traumatic event experienced by a participant. For more information on safety tools, in Chapter 13.

There is a need for more research regarding the ways in which TA-RPG groups can support individuals with a history of trauma. Anecdotal evidence, alongside data from pilot research focusing on TA-RPG groups among military veterans, identified common treatment goals, such as developing appropriate trust, increasing cognitive flexibility, engaging in valued hobbies, improving conflict resolution, and enhancing interpersonal skills (Battles & Quinlan, 2021; Kilmer, 2020; Kilmer & Kilmer, 2018; Roy, 2019).

The utilization of a fictional environment in TA-RPGs creates opportunities for participants to practice interpersonal interaction and to observe the behaviors of others when faced with experiences not typically encountered in a therapeutic setting. The collaborative nature of TTRPGs can support group cohesion. Additionally, participants may be more willing to discuss the hopes and challenges of their characters, as those characters are a step removed from themselves. Further, the game-based setting can support normalization of play, allowing participants to practice creative and flexible thinking with a reduced fear of failure.

A Note on TTRPG Combat and Trauma Replication in TA-RPG Groups

Many TTRPG systems include opportunities for combat and narratives focused on war. These should not necessarily be avoided among individuals with a history of combat-related trauma (e.g., military combat veterans), but should be approached mindfully. Expectations around combat should be discussed with participants prior to the group, and the facilitator should be aware of the participant's boundaries and requests around game content. In the experience of the authors, many combat veterans have expressed appreciation toward opportunities to engage in vicarious simulations of high-fantasy combat. In such instances, the facilitator could increase or decrease the experience of pressure and danger through the tone of their storytelling and through explicit communication. Such encounters allowed participants to observe and better understand how other group members would function in stressful situations, which aided them in developing appropriate trust and group cohesion. Facilitators should be mindful to avoid replicating traumatic content within combat scenarios. For example, a facilitator may want to avoid presenting a scenario where a character becomes trapped under a pile of rubble if there is an individual who experienced a traumatic event in which they were trapped under rubble when a building was bombed. Further, when working with military veterans from a specific era, the facilitator should be aware of common traumatic experiences among that population, for example, improvised explosive devices (IEDs) among veterans of Operation Iraqi Freedom (OIF) and Operation Enduring Freedom (OEF). Finally, facilitators should always approach these experiences from a stance of cultural humility, demonstrating transparency of their knowledge (or lack thereof) and asking participants about their experiences and preferences (Lane, 2019).

Depressive Disorders

Individuals experiencing a depressive episode typically suffer from intense and persistent feelings of sadness or the inability to feel pleasure, as well as changes to their sleep and eating behaviors (APA, 2022; WHO, 2019). They also commonly experience low self-esteem, feelings of worthlessness, and social isolation, which can exacerbate symptoms. During a depressive episode, individuals may lose interest in or not have the energy for valued hobbies or work, further isolating them from peers and reducing exposure to pleasurable stimuli. Psychological intervention for depression often focuses on increasing activity and structure, increasing connection with others, and challenging maladaptive thought patterns that reinforce depressive symptoms (Ekers et al., 2008). Common treatment goals for individuals experiencing depression include identifying and increasing engagement in valued activities, improving connection with others, and increasing their self-esteem.

TA-RPGs create opportunities for individuals experiencing depression to participate in an activity with others at regularly scheduled intervals. This can support the addition of structure to their routine and support mood through behavioral activation. Additionally, through a collaborative and team-focused game, participants are able to observe their impact on both the game world and others around the table, supporting the growth of self-esteem.

Conclusions

Though the experiences and goals discussed in this chapter are not applicable to every individual, there is a commonality among the recommended approach for TA-RPG facilitators working with any population. The facilitator should understand common histories and context, and approach this work from a place of cultural humility. Inherent across both of these recommendations is an underlying respect for the participant and their autonomy, and a prioritization of the relationship between facilitator and participant.

References

American Psychiatric Association. (2022). *Diagnostic and statistical manual of mental disorders* (5th ed., text rev.). Author. https://doi.org/10.1176/appi. books.9780890425787

Arneson, D., & Gygax, G. (1974). *Dungeons & dragons*. TSR.

Barnard-Brak, L., Lechtenberger, D., & Lan, W. Y. (2010). Accommodation strategies of college students with disabilities. *Qualitative Report, 15*(2), 411–429.

Battles, A., & Quinlan, T. (2021, August 12). *Program evaluation of a TA-RPG group therapy with veterans*. In J. N. Kilmer (Chair), Rolling for recovery: Therapeutic applications of tabletop role playing games [Symposium]. American Psychological Association Convention, Online. https://irp.cdn-website.com/a5ea5d51/files/uploaded/APA2021-on-demand-index.pdf

Bauminger, N., & Kasari, C. (2000). Loneliness and friendship in high-functioning children with autism. *Child Development, 71*(2), 447–456.

Bauminger, N., Shulman, C., & Agam, G. (2003). Peer interaction and loneliness in high-functioning children with autism. *Journal of Autism and Developmental Disorders, 33*(5), 489–507.

Bemak, F., & Chung, R. C. Y. (2018). Race dialogues in group psychotherapy: Key issues in training and practice. *International Journal of Group Psychotherapy, 69*(2), 172–191. https://doi.org/10.1080/00207284.2018.1498743

Blackmoore, S., Sullivan, P. K., Turner, L., Balsera, L., Bushyager, M., & Lagace, S. (2019). *Fate of cthulhu*. Evil Hat Productions.

Canu, W. H., & Carlson, G. L. (2003). Differences in heterosocial behavior and outcomes of ADHD-symptomatic subtypes in a college sample. *Journal of Attention Disorders, 6*(3), 123–133. https://doi.org/10.1177/108705470300600304

Caye, A., Swanson, J. M., Coghill, D., & Rohde, L. A. (2019). Treatment strategies for ADHD: An evidence-based guide to select optimal treatment. *Molecular Psychiatry, 24*(3), 390–408.

Cook, A., Ogden, J., & Winstone, N. (2018). Friendship motivations, challenges and the role of masking for girls with autism in contrasting school settings. *European Journal of Special Needs Education, 33*(3), 302–315. https://doi.org/10.1080/08856257.2017.1312797

de Haan, D., Vriens-van Hoogdalem, A. G., Zeijlmans, K., & Boom, J. (2021). Metacommunication in social pretend play: Two dimensions. *International Journal of Early Years Education, 29*(4), 405–419. https://doi.org/10.1080/09669760.2020.1778451

Dhar, P. (2020, November 3). It's time for fantasy fiction and role-playing games to shed their racist history. *The Guardian*. Retrieved June 2, 2022, from www.theguardian.com/games/2020/nov/03/racism-fantasy-fiction-role-playing-games

Douglas, S., & Stirling, L. (2012). Metacommunication, social pretend play and children with autism. *Australasian Journal of Early Childhood, 37*(4), 34–43. https://doi.org/10.1177/183693911203700406

Ekers, D., Richards, D., & Gilbody, S. (2008). A meta-analysis of randomized trials of behavioural treatment of depression. *Psychological Medicine, 38*(5), 611–623. https://doi.org/10.1017/S0033291707001614

Fimi, D. (2022, February 10). Was Tolkien really racist? *The Conversation.* Retrieved June 1, 2022, from https://theconversation.com/was-tolkien-really-racist-108227

Foa, E., Hembree, E., & Rothbaum, B. O. (2007). *Prolonged exposure therapy for PTSD: Emotional processing of traumatic experiences therapist guide.* Oxford University Press.

Garcia, A. (2017). Privilege, power, and Dungeons & Dragons: How systems shape racial and gender identities in tabletop role-playing games. *Mind, Culture, and Activity, 24*(3), 232–246. https://doi.org/10.1080/10749039.2017.1293691

Gygax, G. (1978). *Players handbook.* TSR Games.

Hackett, R. A., Steptoe, A., & Jackson, S. E. (2019). Sex discrimination and mental health in women: A prospective analysis. *Health Psychology, 38*(11), 1014–1024. https://doi.org/10.1037/hea0000796

Hanson, J. (2005). Should your lips be zipped? How therapist self-disclosure and non-disclosure affects clients. *Counselling and Psychotherapy Research, 5*(2), 96–104. https://doi.org/10.1080/17441690500226658

Hays, P. A. (2008). *Addressing cultural complexities in practice: Assessment, diagnosis, and therapy.* American Psychological Association.

Hull, L., Petrides, K. V., & Mandy, W. (2021). Cognitive predictors of self-reported camouflaging in autistic adolescents. *Autism Research, 14*(3), 523–532. https://doi.org/10.1002/aur.2407

Kato, K. (2019). Employing tabletop role-playing games (TRPGs) in social communication support measures for children and youth with autism spectrum disorder (ASD) in Japan: A hands-on report on the use of leisure activities. *Japanese Journal of Analog Role-Playing Game Studies,* 23–28. https://doi.org/10.14989/jarps_0_23

Keenan, E. K. (2004). From sociocultural categories to socially located relations: Using critical theory in social work practice. *Families in Society, 85*(4), 539–548. https://doi.org/10.1177/104438940408500412

Kilmer, E. D. (2020, July). *Role-playing game therapy in a veteran population* [Presentation]. American Lake VA Medical Center Training Day, Tacoma, WA.

Kilmer, J., & Kilmer, E. D. (2018, July). *Therapeutic benefits of role-playing games* [Address]. Waco VA Community Mental Health Summit, Waco, TX.

Kinnear, S. H., Link, B. G., Ballan, M. S., & Fischbach, R. L. (2015). Understanding the experience of stigma for parents of children with autism spectrum disorder and the role stigma plays in families' lives. *Journal of Autism and Developmental Disorders, 46*(3), 942–953.

Knox, S., & Hill, C. E. (2003). Therapist self-disclosure: Research-based suggestions for practitioners. *Journal of Clinical Psychology, 59*(5), 529–539. https://doi.org/10.1002/jclp.10157

Kretchmer, J. (2020, August 21). *Accessibility in gaming resources.* Retrieved August 13, 2022, from https://docs.google.com/document/d/1ZFSXz-Yva1KZAsP7NblCdkoiQ6RcjxSV2gj98eXusJs/edit

Lane, M. (2019). Understanding cultural humility through the lens of a military culture. *Reflections: Narratives of Professional Helping, 25*(1), 90–100. Retrieved June 16, 2022, from https://reflectionsnarrativesofprofessionalhelping.org/index.php/Reflections/article/view/1754

Magnus, E., & Tøssebro, J. (2014). Negotiating individual accommodation in higher education. *Scandinavian Journal of Disability Research, 16*(4), 316–332. https://doi.org/10.1080/15017419.2012.761156

Maïano, C., Normand, C. L., Salvas, M. C., Moullec, G., & Aimé, A. (2016). Prevalence of school bullying among youth with autism spectrum disorders: A systematic review and meta-analysis. *Autism Research, 9*(6), 601–615. https://doi.org/10.1002/aur.1568

Mays, V. M., & Cochran, S. D. (2001). Mental health correlates of perceived discrimination among lesbian, gay, and bisexual adults in the United States. *American Journal of Public Health, 91*(11), 1869–1876. https://doi.org/1/10.2105/AJPH.91.11.1869

McGonigal, J. (2022). *Imaginable: How to see the future coming and be ready for anything*. Bantam Press.

McMahon, J. M., & Kahn, K. B. (2016). Benevolent racism? The impact of target race on ambivalent sexism. *Group Processes & Intergroup Relations, 19*(2), 169–183. https://doi.org/10.1177/1368430215583153

Miller, D., Rees, J., & Pearson, A. (2021). "Masking is life": Experiences of masking in autistic and nonautistic adults. *Autism in Adulthood, 3*(4), 330–338. https://doi.org/10.1089/aut.2020.0083

Milton, D. E. M. (2012). On the ontological status of autism: The 'double empathy problem.' *Disability & Society, 27*(6), 883–887. https://doi.org/10.1080/09687599.2012.710008

Mueller, A. K., Fuermaier, A., Koerts, J., & Tucha, L. (2012). Stigma in attention deficit hyperactivity disorder. *ADHD Attention Deficit and Hyperactivity Disorders, 4*(3), 101–114. https://doi.org/10.1007/s12402-012-0085-3

Ozier, E. M., Taylor, V. J., & Murphy, M. C. (2019). The cognitive effects of experiencing and observing subtle racial discrimination. *Journal of Social Issues, 75*(4), 1087–1115. https://doi.org/10.1111/josi.12349

Paulson, J. F., Buermeyer, C., & Nelson-Gray, R. O. (2005). Social rejection and ADHD in young adults: An analogue experiment. *Journal of Attention Disorders, 8*(3), 127–135. https://doi.org/10.1177/1087054705277203

Pearson, A., & Rose, K. (2021). A conceptual analysis of autistic masking: Understanding the narrative of stigma and the illusion of choice. *Autism in Adulthood, 3*(1), 52–60. https://doi.org/10.1089/aut.2020.0043

Pelton, M. K., Crawford, H., Robertson, A. E., Rodgers, J., Baron-Cohen, S., & Cassidy, S. (2020). Understanding suicide risk in autistic adults: Comparing the Interpersonal Theory of Suicide in autistic and non-autistic samples. *Journal of Autism and Developmental Disorders, 50*(10), 3620–3637. https://doi.org/10.1007/s10803-020-04393-8

Peterson, J. (2012). *Playing at the world: A history of simulating wars, people and fantastic adventures, from chess to role-playing games*. Unreason Press.

Quinlan, M. M., Bates, B. R., & Angell, M. E. (2012). 'What can I do to help?': Postsecondary students with learning disabilities' perceptions of instructors' classroom accommodations. *Journal of Research in Special Educational Needs, 12*(4), 224–233.

Resick, P. A., Monson, C. M., & Chard, K. M. (2016). *Cognitive processing therapy for PTSD: A comprehensive manual.* Guilford Publications.

Ríos-Salas, V., & Larson, A. (2015). Perceived discrimination, socioeconomic status, and mental health among Latino adolescents in US immigrant families. *Children and Youth Services Review, 56*, 116–125. https://doi.org/10.1016/j.childyouth.2015.07.011

Romano, A. (2020, August 18). Lovecraftian horror—and the racism at its core—explained. *Vox.* Retrieved June 1, 2022, from www.vox.com/culture/21363945/hp-lovecraft-racism-examples-explained-what-is-lovecraftian-weird-fiction

Roy, J. (2019, July 16). VA North Texas group therapy uses storytelling . . . and dragons. *VAntage Point.* Retrieved November 2, 2021, from https://blogs.va.gov/VAntage/62951/va-north-texas-group-therapy-uses-storytelling-and-dragons/

Sadusky, J., & Yarhouse, M. (2020). Cultural humility & gender identity. *Reflections: Narratives of Professional Helping, 26*(2), 107–113.

Sellers, R. M., Copeland-Linder, N., Martin, P. P., & Lewis, R. L. H. (2006). Racial identity matters: The relationship between racial discrimination and psychological functioning in African American adolescents. *Journal of Research on Adolescence, 16*(2), 187–216. https://doi.org/10.1111/j.1532-7795.2006.00128.x

Shapiro, F. (2017). *Eye movement desensitization and reprocessing (EMDR) therapy: Basic principles, protocols, and procedures.* Guilford Publications.

Shkedy, G., Sandoval-Norton, A. H., & Shkedy, D. (2020). The trauma of broad-based inclusion for students with autism. *Humanities and Social Science Research, 3*(2), p1. https://doi.org/10.30560/hssr.v3n2p1

Sjunneson, E. (Ed.). (2019). *Fate accessibility toolkit.* Evil Hat Productions.

Stroes, A. D., Alberts, E. D., & der Meere, J. J. V. (2003). Boys with ADHD in social interaction with a nonfamiliar adult: An observational study. *Journal of the American Academy of Child & Adolescent Psychiatry, 42*(3), 295–302. https://doi.org/10.1097/00004583-200303000-00009

Thompson, S. (2020, August 7). *Combat Wheelchair V2.0. mustangsart.* Retrieved August 13, 2021, from https://drive.google.com/drive/folders/1ysDrH2vqKz6NSGkf3_0WX5tV-Ch_t_N_

Witwer, M. (2016). *Empire of imagination: Gary Gygax and the birth of Dungeons & Dragons.* Bloomsbury.

Wizards RPG Team. (2020). *Tasha's cauldron of everything.* Wizards of the Coast LLC.

World Health Organization. (2019). *International statistical classification of diseases and related health problems* (11th ed.). Retrieved from https://icd.who.int/

Yeager, K. A., & Bauer-Wu, S. (2013). Cultural humility: Essential foundation for clinical researchers. *Applied Nursing Research, 26*(4), 251–256. https://doi.org/10.1016/j.apnr.2013.06.008

Yip, T., Gee, G. C., & Takeuchi, D. T. (2008). Racial discrimination and psychological distress: The impact of ethnic identity and age among immigrant and United States-born Asian adults. *Developmental Psychology, 44*(3), 787–800. https://doi.org/10.1037/0012-1649.44.3.787

Case Conceptualization and Treatment Planning in Therapeutically Applied Role-Playing Games

Therapeutically applied role-playing game (TA-RPG) groups, regardless of setting, are conducted with intentionality. This means group members are participating with the goal of engaging in an activity that will support change and growth, though group participants may have a wide range of goals. Therapeutic game masters (GMs) are encouraged to use the language that will be best understood by the stakeholders they are speaking to. With that in mind, the authors believe that the Core Capacities are great descriptive building blocks that can be easily translated to communicate with participants, parents, administrators, and other stakeholders. Once treatment has begun, clear case conceptualization, documentation, and monitoring are an important aspect of ethical implementation of TA-RPG.

Social Flourishing

"Social skills" and social competence are linked with multiple aspects of physical and mental health for children, adolescents, and adults. Adolescents with attention deficit hyperactivity disorder (ADHD) have greater social skill impairment as well as significantly higher odds of being diagnosed with depression when compared with their peers without ADHD (Blackman et al., 2005). Social skills account for a significant part of the association between ADHD and depression (Simoni, 2016). Autism spectrum disorder (ASD) is associated with challenges in social communication as well as co-occurring mental health difficulties (Ratcliffe et al., 2015). Greater mental health difficulties are associated with increased difficulties in social responsiveness and poorer social skills, with social skills accounting for a significant proportion of the variance in mental health scores (Ratcliffe et al., 2015). In adults, diminished social skills are also related to both physical and mental health problems, resulting in increased stress and loneliness (Segrin, 2019). Those with higher social skills may experience less psychological distress as such skills increase access to social support (Segrin et al., 2016).

DOI: 10.4324/9781003281962-8

The aforementioned research shows how social skills are linked to many positive life outcomes. However, many programs designed to target "social skills" are focused on discrete skills, deficit-based, and designed to increase the participant's ability to display neurotypical social behaviors (Bottema-Beutel et al., 2018). This approach runs the risk of ignoring an individual's experience and prioritizing the neurotypical or cultural majority experience (Milton, 2012). These programs can lack nuance around teaching participants how to learn and adapt to a variety of social settings. There are no universal social rules, and as such, heavily scripted behaviors are unlikely to be flexible enough to offer success in a wide range of areas. Additionally, such scripted instruction can discount the reasons why an individual may be hesitant to engage in "typical" social interactions. Examples include prior negative social experiences, a lack of positive social experiences, or a transition from understanding one set of cultural norms to another (i.e., moving to a new area, transition from military to civilian life). The social flourishing model highlights and supports people's authentic personhood as well as their ability to participate and engage socially in ways consistent with their values (Davis et al., 2020). It is fundamentally respectful and places autonomy as a core value. The goals of the social flourishing model include the ability to cultivate meaningful and rewarding relationships with others, set and negotiate appropriate interpersonal boundaries, establish confidence in social interactions, and enhance self-efficacy. Social flourishing heavily overlaps with and relies on psychological flexibility, a key component of mental and physical health (Kashdan & Rottenberg, 2010).

In deficit-based models, the goal is typically to help the participant "fit in" by minimizing the display of atypical behaviors and increasing the display of discrete behaviors. Deficit models can prioritize the demands of the environment, with a strong focus on encouraging the participant in displaying a list of "socially appropriate" behaviors in limited contexts. Though this may produce the desired behaviors in the short term, some individuals report this process is demoralizing and does not support long-term adaptive behaviors (Cassidy et al., 2018; Mitchell et al., 2021).

As an alternative to deficit models, the social flourishing model works to create a supportive and inclusive environment, support discrete skill building with regard to individual autonomy and interest, and increase social confidence. Instead of placing the full responsibility for change on the individual, the social flourishing model extends further by examining ways in which the social or physical environment can be modified to support the participant's well-being and functioning. Goals are set collaboratively, whenever possible, and take into account the participant's social history and values. With a focus on increasing social confidence, participants are supported in establishing positive experiences with social interaction, while practicing the ways in which they want to relate to others. Though direct instruction of skills can still occur within the social flourishing model, universal treatment approaches and behavioral checklists are discouraged in favor of individualized approaches.

Setting Goals

When setting goals with participants, or identifying the general purpose of a TA-RPG group, it is necessary to ensure the facilitator has the appropriate training and experience to support the group in the process of reaching their goals. Facilitators should be clear about the expectations for the group, consistent with current research. For example, at the time of writing this book, there are no peer-reviewed studies that support TA-RPGs as a direct treatment for posttraumatic stress disorder (PTSD), meaning TA-RPGs should not be introduced as an evidence-based treatment for PTSD. However, there is already a strong body of literature that establishes perceived social connectedness and social competence as predictors of healthy functioning in individuals with PTSD (Frueh et al., 2001; Angel et al., 2018; Flannery, 1990; Platt et al., 2014) Additionally, there is a growing body of research demonstrating the positive social outcomes associated with the use of TA-RPGs (Arenas et al., 2022; Baker et al., 2022; Henrich & Worthington, 2021).

Though there are multiple ways of exploring and establishing goals depending on a group's population and context, we have found that the language of the Core Capacities is clear and easily understood by the majority of stakeholders. The Core Capacities are geared toward supporting social and emotional learning goals, helping individuals build the capacity to connect with others on their own terms, and serve as building blocks that impact an individual's ability to thrive in multiple areas.

Core Capacities

The five Core Capacities were first incorporated into Critical Core, the TA-RPG system developed by Game to Grow as an alternative to traditional deficit-based "social skills" groups. As many of these groups are focused on adherence to discrete behavior expectations rooted in western European, neurotypical norms, the Core Capacities are envisioned not to fit participants into certain molds, but to build an individual's capacity to authentically connect with and truly enjoy other people on one's own terms. The development of the Core Capacities is deeply rooted in the Functional Emotional Assessment Scale (FEAS; Greenspan et al., 2001). The Core Capacities should be viewed as building blocks, capacities that can combine and build with each other for rich outcomes. For example, one study found the use of perspective-taking skills to be linked with more useful and original solutions to a group planning and problem-solving activity (Rubenstein et al., 2019). The potential for participants to develop in each of the Core Capacities is built into tabletop role-playing games (TTRPGs), and this potential is harnessed in TA-RPGs to build social confidence and to support social flourishing.

Core Capacities:

- Regulation
- Collaboration
- Planning
- Perspective
- Pretend Play

Regulation

Regulation refers to the ability to manage excitement and distress (i.e., the autonomic nervous system). This includes both emotional and behavioral management of the body and brain's response to stressors (Shields et al., 1994). The ability to regulate emotions and behavior is associated with perceived social competence as well as academic success (Edossa et al., 2018). The goal of regulation is to keep the brain "online" (i.e., calm) and able to think clearly without sliding into a flight, fight, or freeze response. Though the fight, flight, and freeze responses are natural and adaptive responses in many situations, a low threshold for dysregulation can create excessive distress and prevent the individual from engaging in logical decision-making, listening, and responding. The regulation capacity is the foundational capacity, underlying participants' ability to develop and display all other capacities.

Development of regulation is a complex process, and can be impacted by an individual's internal and external environment. In a given situation, an individual's ability to regulate their emotions is influenced by their prior learning history, current situational demands, and the individual's goals for the interaction (Thompson & Calkins, 1996). The optimal way of regulating emotions is contextual, changing based on the individual's environment and their perceived control over that environment. When working on the regulation capacity within TA-RPG groups, the facilitator should remain aware that currently maladaptive regulation strategies were likely adaptive in a prior learning environment (Thompson & Calkins, 1996) and may continue to serve a function within the individual's life.

Common goals related to Regulation include:

- Managing excitement and stress/distress
- Responding appropriately to frustration

- Delaying gratification
- Dealing with high-pressure situations
- Coping with overwhelming sensory stimulation

Regulation in TA-RPGs

Because TA-RPGs are interpersonal and involve randomizing agents (e.g., dice) in the enactment of a story endowed with collective meaning, they are ripe for building the Regulation capacity. In games like Critical Core that use a 20-sided die to determine outcomes of player decisions, there is both a 5% chance of a result of 20 and a 5% chance of a result of 1, regarded respectively as "critical successes" and "critical failures." In a well-played game, these results often create intense levels of excitement and/or stress. Likewise, the narrative sequencing of the game prompts a need for delay-of-gratification, and when a skilled GM facilitates the experience with narrative pacing and high-stakes drama, participants must engage the Regulation capacity to continue enjoying the experience.

Collaboration

The Core Capacity of Collaboration reflects one's ability to work with others to build something more than the sum of its parts. This Core Capacity reflects the established value of collaboration seen in the literature, as well as the increased emphasis of collaborative work due to changing work norms and organizational infrastructure (Laal et al., 2013). While compromise, cooperation, and collaboration can coexist within a supportive relationship and are not mutually exclusive, the aptly named capacity of Collaboration reflects the way relationship dynamics can vary from those defined by conflict-avoidant compromise to life-enriching relationships defined by mutual joy. Often, when children are struggling to work together, they are told by an authoritative figure that they must "compromise." The implicit request of such a statement is often that each child must give up just enough of their desires with the goal of reducing conflict. While this type of compromise is an important life skill, it poorly reflects the potential of relationships to be mutually beneficial. A "cooperative" relationship, one in which two or more individuals are working together toward a common goal, is beneficial for all involved. Labor is shared, burdens are reduced, and outcomes improve. However, enhancing a relationship from cooperative to "collaborative" further improves the interpersonal dynamic. It becomes one of not only mutual support and sharing, but one in which all parties build upon each other's contributions to create something that would have otherwise been impossible. A moment of intimacy, an inside joke, even a joyous burst of playful antagonism—all are reflections of Collaboration.

Collaborative learning and work can support group cohesion, learning retention, and work quality (Laal et al., 2012).

To engage in true Collaboration, individuals must freely participate (i.e., not coerced or cajoled into "prosocial" interaction) and share authentically. Collaborators freely communicate, relying on verbal and nonverbal affective communication. Building on the capacity for Regulation, collaborators offer their contributions without rigid attachment to outcome or ownership, recognizing the benefits of the group's shared creative potential. They must give and receive feedback as they work together, building positive peer reciprocity as they not only work toward their mutual goal but also strengthen their relationship through supportive communication. Over time, the positive experiences support a deep understanding of the value of connecting and working with others.

Common goals related to Collaboration include:

- Communicating verbally (e.g., making clear requests; giving and receiving feedback)
- Communicating nonverbally (e.g., using affect in back-and-forth communication)
- Interacting positively with peers and authority figures
- Working with others toward a common goal
- Sustained back-and-forth communication

Collaboration in TA-RPGs

At the narrative core of many TTRPGs is an ensemble cast of protagonists with a varied array of skills and abilities. Players control a single character who will face in-game scenarios that rely on a wide range of tactics to overcome. Therapeutic GMs will create in-game obstacles that prompt players to dynamically rely on each other. Any single character will not be capable of overcoming the obstacle alone, and players will be supported to communicate effectively in order to be triumphant. Collaborative successes become moments of shared joy that support future motivation to continue collaborating, and moments of intra-group frustration become opportunities for feedback and repair.

Planning

The Planning capacity includes the ability to think on one's feet and respond adaptively to evolving circumstances. The Planning capacity is focused on the use of logical sequencing, multi-causal thinking, critical reasoning, and decisive action to address problems, make and execute plans, and adapt when situations divert from what is expected. Planning and organizational abilities have been positively linked to school outcomes in adolescents (Langberg et al., 2013). Additionally, planning and goal-setting interventions can support better behavioral and academic outcomes in students (Bruhn et al., 2016; Estrapala & Reed, 2020). To predict future events, an individual must understand cause and effect—that specific events occurring in sequence are likely to cause a specific outcome. However, the planning capacity also supports the recognition that sometimes a sequence of events that has occurred many times before may lead to a different outcome entirely when other variables are introduced. Likewise, built into the Planning capacity is the understanding that just because a specific sequence of events led to a specific outcome in the past, that particular outcome may not always be a product of that same sequence of events. (For example: The bus arrived late when a road closure caused a detour. One may reason that future detours may certainly cause bus delays, but one should also recognize that bus delays can be caused by a multitude of factors.) Even when a realistic goal is set and made into a plan of achievable steps in sequence, built on adept logical reasoning and critical thinking, that plan may not manifest as planned for any number of reasons. Planning is vital for imagining the world or oneself as different from what it currently is, which is necessary for increasing motivation to change and adapt habits (Estrapala & Reed, 2020). To be effective at planning the completion of a goal, individuals must be able to set a measurable and attainable goal, then break that goal down into manageable steps, predict and plan for likely obstacles, set reasonable deadlines, and start work toward the goal. Further, the individual needs to be able to adjust the goal when internal or external variables derail the original plan (i.e., the individual getting sick, or more work unexpectedly being assigned). When evaluating an experience, an individual must have an understanding of various potential causes for a single outcome (multi-causal thinking).

Common goals related to planning include:

- Connecting events through cause and effect and multi-causal thinking
- Using critical thinking
- Using deductive and inductive reasoning
- Setting achievable goals
- Predicting obstacles
- Sticking to a previously made plan
- Adapting plans as circumstances evolve

Planning in TA-RPGs

In TA-RPG work, GMs will place characters in front of complex problems to solve, situations with more than one solution that will require logical sequencing and critical reasoning. An objective as seemingly simple as crossing a rickety bridge over a canyon will prompt players to ponder multiple solutions and ideally prompt use of the Collaboration capacity as well. More complex in-game situations will provide even more fodder for planning, such as the need to reveal to the public that the kingdom's rightful ruler has been replaced by a shape-shifting doppelgänger. Each step in the potential plan will cascade into additional inflection points, relying on a comprehensive ability to predict, plan, and respond. Players must additionally use the Regulation capacity as they either commit to a plan despite adversity or abandon a favored plan as situations evolve.

Perspective

The Perspective capacity includes an individual's ability not only to recognize that others *have* unique thoughts, feelings, desires, experiences, and values different from one's own, but also to identify the complex internal worlds of others, consider them, and adjust behaviors in response. At its most basic level, the Perspective capacity is simple theory of mind, but advancement in the Perspective capacity includes the ability to make informed guesses about the internal states of others based on their unique histories and contexts as well as their affective expression. Before individuals can understand complex or conflicted internal states in others, they must be able to understand their own complex internal worlds and experience themselves being witnessed authentically by others. Understanding how to gather needed information to understand and respond to experiences of others is vital to building meaningful trusting relationships, and is also essential to adequately navigate situations that rely on effective interpersonal communication, such as interactions with family and friends, employers and colleagues, medical providers, and even strangers (e.g., a delivery driver or cashier; Nilsen & Bacso, 2017; Todd et al., 2011; Nilsen & Fecica, 2011).

Common goals related to Perspective include:

- Identifying, considering, and adjusting behavior in response to others' thoughts, feelings, desires, experiences, and values
- Developing appropriate trust
- Understanding the role context plays in influencing perspective
- Understanding and recognizing complex and/or conflicted internal states in self and others
- Recognizing mistaken beliefs in others

Perspective in TA-RPG

The Perspective capacity is instilled into any storytelling activity in which players portray characters. As players engage with their characters, they will develop a unique history and background for them, often called a "backstory." This endowment means that the player and the character have at least different knowledge and experiences. As therapeutic GMs guide players to additionally consider a character's feelings, beliefs, values, etc. (often informed by the character's backstory and individual context), the characters are imbued with even more complex internal worlds. Players are invited to decide how their characters will respond to the in-game situations informed by those aspects, and are encouraged to have their characters evolve in response to new moments in the story, reflecting the real-world way individuals learn, grow, and change.

Pretend Play

The Pretend Play capacity is a synthesis of capacities for symbolic and abstract thinking, imitative and imaginative "make-believe," and a disposition of curiosity and active engagement with the inherent potential of each moment. Play is a vital part of human development, instrumental in the development of social, cognitive, and emotional skills (Milteer et al., 2012). Building on the writing of Brown (2009), the Pretend Play capacity involves the ability to participate fully in an activity with minimal distress and to be so engaged that one loses track of time, de-prioritizes adherence to rules, and experiences a reduction in performance anxiety. This level of engagement is not dissociative; it is a whole-brained state of flow (Nakamura & Csikszentmihalyi, 2014). This capacity also involves the ability to imagine alternate realities informed by our own and to envision divergent futures, to imagine not only the way the world is but also how it could be and to become an active agent of change to make it so. Similar in some respects to simulation training (Gelis et al., 2020; Pilnick et al., 2018), TA-RPG participants are invited to enter into a liminal play-based simulacrum, where they are able to experiment with alternate behaviors and try on new aspects of their identity.

Common goals related to pretend play include:

- Imitating real life
- Imagining alternate realities and different futures
- Interpreting humor
- Practicing skills
- Testing out identities

Pretend Play in TA-RPG

TA-RPGs involve a clear set of rules, guidelines, and participation structures, which provide boundaries and a safe container in which players can engage with minimal distress. Adept therapeutic GMs will recognize that the rules, guidelines, and participation structures are tools to be used selectively to promote participant engagement but that they can also be applied, modified, and ignored selectively to meet player needs. Therapeutic GMs encourage players to lean into the simulated reality co-constructed by the cohort, embrace the whimsy, and lead with their curiosity to make discoveries.

Combining the Blocks

The Core Capacities are foundations on which more complex goals can be built. As mentioned earlier, the Core Capacities are not discrete skills, but can be conceived of as building blocks to higher order goals. Some examples include:

- Conflict Resolution = Regulation + Collaboration + Perspective
- Completing Projects = Regulation + Collaboration + Planning
- Changing Habits = Regulation + Planning + Pretend Play

Communicating With Stakeholders

Any TA-RPG group has multiple stakeholders. Participants, parents or guardians of participants, supervisors or site administrators, or even insurance companies may be a stakeholder or gatekeeper for a TA-RPG group. When speaking with stakeholders and advocating for TA-RPGs, it is important to understand each stakeholder's goals and priorities, and use language that will be best understood by each stakeholder. For example, a ten-year-old participant may be interested in a safe place to learn to play TTRPGs. For this stakeholder, discussing the opportunities for gameplay and character customization would be the most appropriate way to frame expectations. For a parent interested in a group to support their child's social confidence, the priority of conversation should be the opportunity for low stakes social interaction and the social scaffolding provided by TA-RPGs. Administrators and supervisors may benefit from a more technical explanation of how client goals are uniquely addressed through TA-RPG gameplay, or the way in which TA-RPGs may serve as a positive re-introduction into mental health care for treatment-fatigued clients.

Functional Analysis

To be an effective therapeutic GM, facilitators must develop skills around predicting and influencing behavior in ways that support group relationships and respect participant autonomy. Every behavior displayed by a participant, no matter how "annoying" or "maladaptive," has a function (Hayes et al., 2012). Sometimes, the consequences of a behavior do not line up the participant's intentions, or they may go beyond what the intent of the behavior was (Murphy et al., 2019). For example, a participant who is attempting to influence another participant to stop tapping their pencil on the table shouts, "Stop making that noise, you jerk!" Though this may influence the pencil-tapping participant to stop the noise, the form of the behavior (yelling and calling another participant names) is likely to have consequences not intended by the participant. For facilitators to effectively support participants toward their goals, and maintain a safe and supportive group environment, understanding how to identify the "why" of behaviors is essential.

The functional analysis framework typically follows an ABC formula: antecedent, behavior, consequence. The *antecedent* is what prompts the behavior. Though antecedents often have an environmental cue, an individual's experience of the world is translated through their history and understanding of the world. Thus, the antecedent includes both the environmental cue and the internal thoughts, feelings, and memories associated with the cue. As such, not all cues are "equal" for all participants. A tapping pencil may be background noise for some, while for others the sound quickly becomes intolerable. The *behavior* is the action being observed and analyzed. Finally, the *consequences* are the short- and long-term impacts of the behavior. In the pencil-tapping example, the pencil tapping stopped, but there may be immediate and/or long-term damage to the relationship of the participants as a consequence of the behavior.

When the facilitator has an understanding of the antecedents, behaviors, and consequences, they can support the participant in achieving the function of the original behavior with fewer negative consequences (Hayes et al., 2012). When using functional behavior analysis as a way to support adaptive behavior change, it can be tempting to focus on consequences as a way to change behavior. This can be especially salient when working with new individuals (or new behaviors), as there is little opportunity to influence the antecedents prior to observing the behavior. However, intervening in the consequence stage (especially with punishment) may be more likely to suppress the behavior without establishing an adaptive replacement behavior. Using the function of the behavior as a guide, facilitators can support participants in identifying new strategies to meet their needs.

When utilizing functional behavior analysis in TA-RPG groups, there may not be sufficient time to check in with the participant about their intended function, or such explicit communication may be inappropriate because of the participant or setting. This means that facilitators will often need to make assumptions about the function of the behavior. When making assumptions about participant behavior, the facilitator should always *assume the best possible intent consistent with the facts.*

This reduces the likelihood that the facilitator inaccurately assumes an intent of malice, selfishness, or another intent that could damage their relationship with the participant, as well as damage the participant's social confidence and sense of safety in the group. Especially for participants who have a long history of adults or authority figures "assuming the worst," these kinds of assumptions can instill a sense of helplessness in participants that can inhibit movement toward more prosocial behaviors. In cases where the participant has *worse* intentions than assumed by the facilitator, an opportunity can be created for the participant to "try again" in their approach to a particular outcome. Such responses can send the message that the participant is a valued and respected member of the group and allow for the rehearsal of more adaptive behaviors.

Three Dimensions of Capacity Building

In many contexts, when a learner does not exhibit a desired behavior (i.e., they leave a portion of a math assignment blank or refrain from introducing themselves to a new classmate), the common assumption is that the individual lacks the knowledge needed to implement the behavior. While this can be true, relying on this assumption can lead to frustrated facilitators and demoralized participants. Utilizing a functional analysis with the three dimensions of capacity building can help facilitators effectively scaffold their participants. In this section, we build off the three types of deficits identified by DeMatteo et al. (2012), with language adjusted to better fit the social flourishing approach.

The three dimensions of capacity building are:

- Knowledge
- Performance
- Fluency

The Knowledge Dimension

Knowledge is required before an individual can implement a skill or strategy. When a participant has proficiency in the *knowledge* dimension, they understand what the behavior is and when it should typically be utilized. For example, a participant may understand that when one is interested in meeting a new person, they can walk up to them, say "Hello," provide their name, and ask for the name of the other person. If a participant has never had experience or modeling of introductions before, and they do not have the framework for that particular interaction (e.g., scripts, decision trees, etc.), direct instruction can support the growth of the knowledge dimension in that area.

The Performance Dimension

When a participant lacks proficiency in the *performance* dimension, they have knowledge of the skill, but may not feel confident or comfortable displaying the skill. This can be related to prior experience with the behavior (e.g., failure to achieve the intended or appropriate outcome when displaying the behavior) or fear of trying out the behavior for the first time. Participants developing the performance dimension can benefit from encouragement and reinforcement, that is, low stakes, high-reward opportunities to rehearse the skill as they first start to display it within the group. See the sections on affect in Chapter 11 for more information on reinforcement.

The Fluency Dimension

When a participant needs support in the *fluency* dimension, they have both knowledge and comfort performing a skill, but are working on increasing their ease and success rate executing the skill. Participants in this area do not need additional teaching or encouragement, but will benefit from modeling, coaching, and feedback. Often modeling and feedback from non-player characters (NPCs) can be the least intimidating, while positive feedback from other participants can be the most meaningful.

Functional behavior analysis and the three dimensions of capacity building support participants to leverage behaviors that get them closer to their goals. Insight into which dimension needs further development can often be derived from observation of a behavior (or its absence) and contextual factors surrounding the behavior.

For example, if a participant is asked what their character does next in a combat sequence and they stare down at their character sheet silently, this could be a knowledge or performance deficit. If the facilitator is aware that the participant is familiar with their character and their moves, and has played TTRPGs before, the facilitator may hypothesize that the player has a performance deficit. The player has the knowledge needed to complete their turn, but they may not feel comfortable displaying the behavior (describing their character's actions) in the current context. The facilitator should examine the environment for further possible contributions to the antecedents driving this behavior. Did combat take an unexpected turn and the player needs more time to think of their answer? Did another player scoff at their choice the last time they took a turn? If all the other players spoke in their character's voice to describe their actions, this player may need encouragement to participate or reassurance that they do not have to use a special voice for their character right now. Understanding where the player is on the dimensions of capacity building and the context that contributes to their current functioning will allow the facilitator to appropriately scaffold the participant to improve their skill development.

Case Conceptualization and Treatment Planning

When developing a treatment plan, it is important to conceptualize the goals for the intervention with a particular individual, as well as understand the context in which the treatment is occurring. Further, this conceptualization should be updated in accordance with participant and group progress, contextual changes, and stated goals. We recommend having a central document in which the following areas are regularly updated with the date of each update. This is valuable for check-ins with participants and parents, as well as an overview for the facilitator as they plan sessions or encounters. These areas can be folded into existing treatment plans and treatment notes, or be kept as a separate document.

Participant Strengths

What aptitudes, talents, or skills does the participant currently possess? Are they great at making quick decisions during fast-paced games? Do they enjoy reading and remembering complex rulesets? Do they persist at challenges they find interesting? When identifying participant strengths, it is valuable to seek information on strengths from multiple perspectives and contexts. If the participant struggles to identify strengths related to home, work, or school environments, they may be able to identify strengths related to hobby environments.

Participant Challenges

What areas cause distress in the participant's current life? Challenges are often related to current goals—a participant who describes feeling "out of control" of their emotions may have goals related to emotional regulation or insight.

Context of Treatment

Where, how, and why is this intervention happening? Is the participant excited about TA-RPGs, or are they participating reluctantly? Is the group an in-person group or a virtual group? Does the group happen right after school or work? The context of the group can impact participants' ability to engage and willingness to participate.

Accommodations

Are there any supports or changes to the group environment that can increase the participant's ability to engage? Accommodations should be designed to increase the ability for participants to take part in the group without reducing their autonomy. For example, a participant who is visually impaired may choose to use braille dice or a virtual dice roller to allow them to roll their own dice. More information about accommodations can be found in Chapter 7.

Participant Goals

What is the participant hoping to achieve or develop in this group? Participants often have game- and group-related goals. A participant may want to learn more about how to play a TTRPG and/or how to self-advocate in social situations. Participants may also not have clearly defined goals.

Parent/Treatment Team Goals

Where applicable, the facilitator should consider the treatment goals of a participant's parent, treatment team, or other stakeholder. Parents and treatment teams may have explicit treatment goals for the participant.

Facilitator Goals

As the facilitator works with the participant and the group, the facilitator may also develop treatment goals for the participant. These goals typically heavily overlap with the participant's challenges and goals, and may articulate a series of goals toward the participant's own goals. For example, if a participant's goal is to "make friends," the facilitator may identify goals related to collaboration and perspective that would further support the participant's goal to develop friendships with peers.

Facilitator Interventions

Though not every intervention utilized by the facilitator should be documented in this case conceptualization, themes or particularly successful interventions should be noted to inform future planning.

Observed Participant Growth

Participant progress, especially when in-line with identified goals, should be recorded. Often a brief narrative description of the events and the goals or Core Capacities with which they relate is a beneficial way to record progress in a way that can be used later in treatment planning and as examples for stakeholders.

Support Provided by the Group

TA-RPGs are group interventions, and making note of the group interactions is a necessary part of treatment planning and observing progress. Noting the frequency of supportive processes, as well as noting how group members offer support, can provide insight into both group and individual development. More information about group development can be found in Chapter 9.

Support Provided to the Group

In addition to noting the support provided by the group, observing the participant's willingness to support other members can provide valuable information into the participant's connection with group members and their progress toward interpersonal goals.

Recommendations/Next Steps

The recommendations for treatment and next steps can include recommendations for in-game changes, supports, or challenges, as well as interventions outside of the group.

Player Characters and Treatment Planning

While the character itself is a fictional person existing in a simulated world, the character must also be deconstructed onto a character sheet to accommodate the rules of the TTRPG being played. Character sheets typically contain necessary information such as abilities (e.g., physical strength, knowledge, and charisma) and skills (e.g., diplomacy or stealth), as well as additional information such as personality traits, physical characteristics, and background/backstory information. Often, a character sheet is an imperfect approximation of the client's conceptualization of the character.

The use of a character is a valuable therapeutic tool in TA-RPG. Both the process and the final product of character creation can reveal much about a client's perception of themselves, others, and the world around them. Commonly, clients are moved to create a character they believe reflects who they currently are (albeit in a fantasy setting), an "ideal self" character (i.e., what the player believes to be the "best" version of themselves), or a "feared self" character (i.e., someone they are afraid of becoming). Clients with more TTRPG experience may be increasingly interested in creating characters that are discrepant from their current selves, complete with traits they would like to develop or improve upon. In such cases, clients may express more insight into how they hope to explicitly use their character to address their treatment goals. Though primarily focused on video game avatars, some research has found that playing an avatar with characteristics different from oneself can change an individual's behavior in real life (Yee et al., 2009). Regardless of the degree of similarity between clients and their character, it is the client who drives the character through the narrative of each session. Thus, their typical patterns of behavior toward themselves, others, and the world are inherently preserved and remain demonstrably present in their character's behavior.

At times, a TA-RPG provider may be unable to engage in a thorough intake session with the client, or the client may struggle to formulate their treatment goals. In such cases, a player's character sheet can provide insight into the client for both the therapist and the client. Although character sheets should not be used as a diagnostic tool, they can be utilized to formulate working hypotheses around a client's self-image and potential therapeutic goals. As an example, consider the case of Tara:

> Prior to the group, the facilitator had the opportunity to consult with Tara's individual provider, but did not meet with her for a separate intake. Tara's provider shared she struggled with making friends at school, experienced bullying, and had a recent history of trauma. In this group, participants selected from several prepared pre-made character sheets, and were invited to fill in the name, physical characteristics, and background information such as personality traits, bonds, ideals, flaws. Tara described her character as having no friends, with the goal to destroy the world and re-make it with only her character present. She listed her character's personality trait in one word—"angry," with the flaw noted as "depressed." Tara's character description was consistent with the challenges Tara's individual provider reported—and led the facilitator to hypothesize that Tara may have a negative self-image and be likely to engage in rejecting behavior to others to mitigate fears and expectations around rejection.

Once hypotheses have been formed, it may be prudent for the therapist to collaboratively discuss these insights with the client to maintain healthy client–therapist alignment and appropriate expectations for treatment. As with any working hypotheses, they will be refined and adjusted over time as the therapist gathers new data about the client and their experience. Further, similar to character sheets, these hypotheses should shift over time, as both the client and their character grow and develop new skills and beliefs.

A Note on Risk Assessment and Character Creation

The Game to Grow Method of TA-RPGs does not include a formal risk assessment process or protocol. However, in any clinical setting, clients may present with, or be at risk for, self-harm and/or suicidal behaviors. As with any treatment, clinical judgment should be used to decide when to formally assess risk. A client's description of their character or their character's behavior may be indications of possible risk and should be viewed as such.

A Note on "Evil" Characters

Many TTRPG systems include a "character alignment" mechanic as part of the character creation process. This mechanic typically has a two-pronged axis, with "chaotic" to "lawful" on one axis and "good" to "evil" on the other. This mechanic is typically used to help describe how predictable (the chaotic/lawful axis) and prosocial (the evil/good axis) characters will act. It often functions in two ways: as a descriptor/reflection of character action (e.g., the character stole from an orphanage so therefore they are "evil") and a structured tool to classify characters that informs player decisions (e.g., the character is "evil" so therefore they would steal from an orphanage). In either context, alignment can change over time and should not be considered a binding contract for character action. Having character alignment as an explicit mechanic is not always valuable for therapeutic growth, so TA-RPG facilitators should decide prior to running a group whether they will include the mechanic and how comfortable they are running a game wherein one or more players choose to play a character with an evil alignment.

Depending on the needs of the group, it may be either prudent or contraindicated to allow evil characters. In the worst cases, such an allowance can unintentionally license one or more players to engage in wantonly destructive and antisocial behaviors within the game and create an unsafe space for other players. A player with unclear expectations about group goals and purpose, or one who has a tendency to push others away before they can be rejected, is likely to engage in significant boundary violations through their character. In this context, the safety of the group and the therapeutic potential of a neutral starting character likely outweigh the potential benefits of player autonomy in character alignment choice.

However, when the participant's decision to play a character that is labeled as "evil," is instead tied to negative self-worth/self-loathing, it may provide a valuable therapeutic opportunity. The conscious choice to play an evil character is often tied to intentional treatment goals (e.g., self-esteem, communication, social connection, insight). Other times, selecting an evil-aligned character may be an unconscious choice on the part of the player. If their character is described as "evil" but engages in prosocial behavior, the distinction between the characters expected and actual actions can create space for re-examination of the participant's own self-image and provides ample opportunities to challenge the player's maladaptive beliefs about their self-worth. Thus, eliminating a client's agency to choose their character's alignment can also eliminate potentially powerful interventions. Regardless, allowing clients to play evil characters should not entail the elimination of in-game consequences for antisocial or otherwise "evil" actions. Such consequences help to illustrate similar potential real-world consequences, serve as experiential learning opportunities, and help to maintain in-game boundaries.

Character Types

Because narrative transference and aesthetic distance are foundations of the Game to Grow Method, the way a player relates to their character is an important concept for therapeutic GMs to understand and leverage. Players may not engage in character creation and character portrayal with therapeutic intent, but the way a player plays their character can regardless be interpreted as at least partial reflections of their goals and needs. The character types outlined in the following, inspired by the writings of Bowman (2010), are an imperfect set of archetypes that can assist case conceptualization and treatment planning. The typology is not entirely discrete. Various character aspects and role-play choices will align with more than one of the categories. Understanding how a player's character relates to their explicit or implicit goals and reflects their lived experience may guide the session design process and the degree to which aesthetic distance is leveraged to support player growth through identification with their character.

Looking-Glass Character

A character that is created or role-played with similar motivations, attitudes, and demeanor as the player is considered a "looking-glass character"; a reference to Alice's journey into Wonderland where she enters a fantastical world but retains her core fundamental attributes. Looking glass characters will naturally have skills, abilities, and physical attributes that the player does not (e.g., access to magic), often based on the specific TTRPG game system. However, the act of role-play and associated character motivations will largely be based on the participant's own self-concept. Sometimes, these characters are a reflection of inexperience with TTRPGs and will evolve as players become more familiar with the openness of narrative exploration. Other times, the players intentionally want to create a character like themselves.

Amplified-Self Character

An amplified-self character is one whose attitudes, motivations, and aspects are fundamentally similar to their own lived experience, only with an attribute amplified. The amplified attribute may be one regarded as positive or maladaptive. As an example, a participant who may be described in their out-of-game context as "impulsive" may create or role-play a character whose impulsivity is amplified. The character may routinely jump into action without planning or react suddenly to new situations without thinking. In such a case, the impulsivity of the character is an amplified aspect that may be a valuable concept for processing.

Similarly, an individual with a prosocial demeanor, or one with personal attributes regarded positively, may likewise amplify those aspects in their character. Amplification of these self-concepts creates opportunities for insight. A participant who is routinely in service of others, who is constantly helping and conceding their interest to prioritize others', may create or role-play a helper character that amplifies these attributes. Because the helper characters may be regarded as positive and prosocial, benefitting the group and promoting in-game success, the GM may be inclined to reinforce the character portrayal, though they may respond differently depending on the individual participant goals. If the player struggles with self-advocacy, deferring or acquiescing to others in their own life in a way that contradicts their goals and their values, the GM may selectively encourage or disincentivize the portrayal in the game. The GM may intentionally design an encounter where their character must take initiative and lead the group instead of acting in service to the others.

Aspirational Character

Many players, especially when guided by a therapist to do so, will create aspirational characters with traits the participant would like to possess, or exhibit more. These traits may include the strength, intellect, or abilities of the character as portrayed on the character sheet, or be reflected in the portrayal of the character (e.g., confidence, social acclaim, willingness to set boundaries). Understanding which attributes of a player's character are aspirational in nature will guide a therapeutic GM to selectively reinforce their positive self-concept. If a participant struggles to have a positive social life and creates or portrays their character as a widely respected and celebrated war hero, the GM may interpret this portrayal as aspirational and choose to build encounters so that the participant internalizes the sense of social confidence. The story may involve opportunities for the character to be positively regarded so that the player can experience the positive regard of others for therapeutic impact.

Shadow Character

Character creation and role-play is an opportunity for players to explore parts of their identity, either intentionally or as a reflection of subconscious phenomena, that they might otherwise have difficulty portraying. Some players may choose to include aspects into their character that they may be personally exploring, hiding, or otherwise less comfortable expressing. These "shadow" aspects may be a reflection of a player's discomfort with but willingness to explore aspects of their own identity. Aspects explored through a shadow character are not necessarily problematic. For example, players may choose to explore concepts of gender expression through their character, choosing to play characters of other genders to "try on" the identity. Similarly, self-concepts that may prompt the player's shame-humiliation may be intentionally or unintentionally portrayed in their character. A player who experiences pressure to be "professional" or "mature" in their everyday life may portray their character as a youthful, naive, and mischievous prankster that playfully disrupts the intentions of others.

The category in which a therapeutic GM interprets a character's portrayal of their character will inform how they allow the story to respond. The same character portrayal performed by different players may be responded to differently depending on the GM's interpretation. A player who is portraying their character as brash and unapologetic, threatening and otherwise acting aggressively toward NPCs, could be any of the four character types. For a player who is naturally blunt and aggressive, this may be a looking-glass portrayal or an amplified-self character. The GM may respond to this interpretation by designing in-game encounters that guide the player toward insights that this behavior may not serve their goals, or help provide opportunities for more prosocial interactions. A player who is naturally meek and overly apologetic may be portraying the same behavior as an aspirational character or a shadow character. Depending on the interpretation, the GM may overtly celebrate or implicitly reward the portrayal, encouraging the player to practice a new way of interacting with their environment that may not be literally ideal for real-world replication, but one that is at its essence aligned with the player's therapeutic goals of confidence building and comfort taking up space.

Outcome Monitoring

Monitoring client progress in order to adapt treatment as appropriate is considered an important part of evidence-based practice for good reason (Dyer et al., 2016). The documented benefits of routine monitoring of client progress include improved outcomes, risk identification, reduced dropout rate, and an increased rate of symptom reduction (Gondek et al., 2016; Harmon et al., 2005; Percevic et al., 2004; Shimokawa et al., 2010).

Formal monitoring of participant progress, followed by feedback on such progress to clients (and parents when applicable), can increase client buy-in to treatment as well as increase rapport (Boswell et al., 2015; Youn et al., 2012). This can be particularly helpful with more novel interventions, such as when participants are unfamiliar with TA-RPGs.

Though many outcome measures can be expensive and time-consuming, there are options available that are free for non-commercial purposes, such as the Strengths and Difficulties Questionnaire (Goodman, 2001). This is a short measure with forms for ages three to adult, and has been validated in multiple languages. It is a screening measure that touches on multiple areas of a client's life that may be impacted by TA-RPGs and takes only a few minutes to complete. If a facilitator's setting or practice uses outcome motoring measures that fit well with common client goals in their setting, these measures may be appropriate for your TA-RPG groups as well.

In addition to standardized measures, the facilitator should regularly update their case conceptualization and track progress on a treatment plan document, such as the one outlined in the previous section. Such methods of tracking allow for the recording of narrative descriptions, participant comments, and feedback that are not captured by most standardized measures.

Documentation

Session documentation is an important part of outcome monitoring, and formal session documentation is required in many settings. Progress notes will typically include a brief mention of relevant narrative game content, in addition to progress on identified treatment goals, participant responses, and other notable content. When formulating documentation, the check-out questions outlined in Chapter 10 are a great starting point to address the necessary documentation components.

The type of documentation appropriate for each session depends on the group and setting type. Therapeutic social skills groups in many community settings may not require formal, individualized notes for each participant for each session, while counseling groups will typically require individual notes to comply with insurance, agency, and practice guidelines. TA-RPG groups can be easily documented within existing agency or practice templates and guidelines. Following is an example progress note from a psychotherapy group conducted in a large hospital, consistent with the agency's documentation standards. When formal documentation is not required, we still recommend documentation at a group level, with regular updates for each participant's case conceptualization document.

Group Name: Depression and Dragons
Length: 120 minutes
CPT Code: 90853
Number of Participants: 4
Methodology: Interact, process/discuss, and handouts
Facilitator: TA-RPG Facilitator Name, Credentials
CONTENT:
During the current session, group members met, via telecommunication software, to practice target skills through therapeutic application of the role-playing game, Dungeons and Dragons. Clients were introduced to vicarious scenarios designed to elicit social interaction and skills training, teamwork, perspective taking, and problem solving. During these interactions, members took turns expressing their insight into their character's thoughts and behaviors. Within the session's story, the group worked to rescue a townsperson that was kidnapped by werewolves during the first session. Group members took turns solving problems and supporting each other through a series of trials including tracking the werewolves, assisting each other in their actions, negotiating with non-player characters, and practicing effective communication and planning among each other.

Time was dedicated at the end of the group for processing. Questions were posed to each member regarding their contributions to the group dynamic. Specifically, the clients were asked to name one thing their characters learned in their current adventure. Answers included: "I can interact with the world in more ways than I realized," "I made friends that I can trust," and "I saw how impulsivity impacts others." Additionally, each group member took turns highlighting important/helpful choices and actions other group members took throughout the adventure.

Participants also reflected that engaging in this group consistently improves their mood for the day. Participants and clinician explored some of the possible mechanics of this, including positive social interaction, humor, increased insight, and feelings of accomplishment. Participants were challenged to engage in something that makes them feel positive this week. Ideas they produced included completing a chore, watching funny memes online, and calling a loved one.

Group members demonstrated increased collaboration and willingness to make personal sacrifices for the sake of other individuals and the team as a whole. Several group members noted they felt safe while exploring the dangers of the werewolves' lair due to their trust in their fellow group members.

ASSESSMENT:

Participant was present and participated in group today. Participant appeared to be oriented to date, place, and time.

Participant did not endorse suicidal/homicidal thoughts, plans, or intent.

There were no indications of imminent risk in the participant's presentation.

The participant was casually dressed with unremarkable hygiene and grooming. The participant actively engaged in today's group. Mood appeared generally stable; affect and behavior were within normal limits.

DIAGNOSIS: F33.1 Major Depressive Disorder, Recurrent, Moderate

PLAN: Participant will continue on in the Depression and Dragons group, to support goals of increased positive interactions with others and comfort articulating internal experiences.

Check-In Sessions

Check-in sessions with participants and parents (where applicable) are an excellent opportunity to collaboratively evaluate progress toward goals, set expectations, and receive feedback on the TA-RPG group. These check-ins should happen on a regular basis, and typically last 30 minutes. For most settings, we recommend one 30-minute check-in per ten weeks of weekly services; however, this should be adjusted based on participant needs, population, and setting.

Participant Check-In Sessions

Participant check-ins allow the participant and facilitator to discuss progress thus far in group, update treatment goals, and clarify treatment expectations as needed. These should be collaborative processes between facilitator and participant. For some adolescent participants, parent check-in sessions alone may be more appropriate than a joint or participant check-in session. This should be determined by factors such as setting, clinical concerns, and participant preference.

Parent Check-In Sessions

When appropriate for adolescent participants, parent check-in sessions can be a valuable tool for supporting participants in TA-RPGs. These sessions allow the facilitator to answer questions parents have about TA-RPGs and their child's particular group, the progress the facilitator has seen and facilitated within the group, and recommended next steps.

Collaboration With Other Treatment Providers

As with any other therapeutic interventions, facilitators may consult or collaborate with a participant's other treatment providers to ensure the client is receiving the best care. When communicating with other treatment providers, the facilitator should consider the information they need to provide, as well as the information they want to receive from the provider. Though the specifics will depend on the participant, provider type, and setting, there are several general areas of information that will be relevant for most treatment teams.

Information to Provide

Basic information about the goals and structure of TTRPGs and TA-RPGs can support the consulted provider in effectively communicating about the TA-RPG group with the participant and integrating the group more effectively in the participant's treatment plan. Interventions or coping strategies that have been effective in the participant's TA-RPG group and will generalize to other settings should also be shared with the consulted provider. Finally, information about goals and observed or reported progress should be shared.

Information to Solicit

Collecting information related to participant goals, coping strategies, stressors, and potential roadblocks can support the facilitator's case conceptualization, treatment planning, and in-group support of the participant.

Termination and Beyond

When a client graduates from a TA-RPG group, they walk away with the ability to engage in a new hobby. The transition from TA-RPG group to recreational TTRPG group can be an immensely rewarding one. Recreational TTRPG groups provide a semi-structured social space that may be less overwhelming to individuals with recently developed or reclaimed social skills than a less structured event such as a bar, coffee shop, or party. Such a hobby can also support auxiliary goals, such as making new friends or meeting new people. Further, recreational TTRPG groups can continue to support goals related to behavioral activation, social engagement, schedule consistency, and accountability.

Depending on the client's prior experience with TTRPGs, the facilitator should discuss the differences between a TA-RPG group and a recreational TTRPG group. TTRPGs played in a social setting may not be played with the same intentionality, and there may be less patience afforded to players or characters that cause distress to others at the table. Additionally, there will not be the same expectations regarding confidentiality or group processing. Finally, unless playing within a game with standardized rules (such as D&D Adventurers League), participants should expect the rules may change between groups.

Depending on the goals of the group, the process of finding a recreational TTRPG group that is a good fit can be an important topic to discuss. Participants may have beliefs that this group is the "only" group that will really work for them. It may be beneficial to explore these beliefs by having clients try out several different recreational TTRPG groups before the final session. The group's own forming process, especially if it was a particularly rocky one, may be a great way to highlight the nonlinear process of group formation and getting to know new people.

References

Angel, C. M., Smith, B. P., Pinter, J. M., Young, B. B., Armstrong, N. J., Quinn, J. P., . . ., & Erwin, M. S. (2018). Team Red, White & Blue: A community-based model for harnessing positive social networks to enhance enrichment outcomes in military veterans reintegrating to civilian life. *Translational Behavioral Medicine*, *8*(4), 554–564. https://doi.org/10.1093/tbm/iby050

Arenas, D. L., Viduani, A., & Araujo, R. B. (2022). Therapeutic use of role-playing game (RPG) in mental health: A scoping review. *Simulation & Gaming*, *53*(3), 285–311. https://doi.org/10.1177/10468781211073720

Baker, I. S., Turner, I. J., & Kotera, Y. (2022). Role-play games (RPGs) for mental health (Why not?): Roll for initiative. *International Journal of Mental Health and Addiction*, 1–9. https://doi.org/10.1007/s11469-022-00832-y

Blackman, G. L., Ostrander, R., & Herman, K. C. (2005). Children with ADHD and depression: A multisource, multimethod assessment of clinical, social, and academic functioning. *Journal of Attention Disorders*, *8*(4), 195–207. https://doi.org/10.1177/1087054705278777

Boswell, J. F., Kraus, D. R., Miller, S. D., & Lambert, M. J. (2015). Implementing routine outcome monitoring in clinical practice: Benefits, challenges, and solutions. *Psychotherapy Research*, *25*(1), 6–19. https://doi.org/10.1080/10503 307.2013.817696

Bottema-Beutel, K., Park, H., & Kim, S. Y. (2018). Commentary on social skills training curricula for individuals with ASD: Social interaction, authenticity, and stigma. *Journal of Autism and Developmental Disorders, 48*(3), 953–964. https://doi.org/10.1007/s10803-017-3400-10

Bowman, S. L. (2010). *The functions of role-playing games: How participants create community, solve problems and explore identity.* McFarland.

Brown, S. L. (2009). *Play: How it shapes the brain, opens the imagination, and invigorates the soul.* Penguin.

Bruhn, A. L., McDaniel, S. C., Fernando, J., & Troughton, L. (2016). Goal-setting interventions for students with behavior problems: A systematic review. *Behavioral Disorders, 41*(2), 107–121. https://doi.org/10.17988/0198-7429-41.2.107

Cassidy, S., Bradley, L., Shaw, R., & Baron-Cohen, S. (2018). Risk markers for suicidality in autistic adults. *Molecular Autism, 9*(1), 42. https://doi.org/10.1186/s13229-018-0226-4

Davis, A., Johns, A., & Spielmann, V. (2020, November 9). *Development with dice: From core deficit to critical capacities* [Conference Session]. The 24th Annual International DIRFLOORTIME® Conference: Floortime All the Time and Everywhere.

DeMatteo, F. J., Arter, P. S., Sworen-Parise, C., Fasciana, M., & Paulhamus, M. A. (2012). Social skills training for young adults with autism spectrum disorder: Overview and implications for practice. *National Teacher Education Journal, 5*(4), 57–65.

Dyer, K., Hooke, G. R., & Page, A. C. (2016). Effects of providing domain specific progress monitoring and feedback to therapists and patients on outcome. *Psychotherapy Research, 26*(3), 297–306. https://doi.org/10.1080/10503307.2014.983207

Edossa, A. K., Schroeders, U., Weinert, S., & Artelt, C. (2018). The development of emotional and behavioral self-regulation and their effects on academic achievement in childhood. *International Journal of Behavioral Development, 42*(2), 192–202. https://doi.org/10.1177/0165025416687412

Estrapala, S., & Reed, D. K. (2020). Goal-setting instruction: A step-by-step guide for high school students. *Intervention in School and Clinic, 55*(5), 286–293. https://doi.org/10.1177/1053451219881717

Flannery, Jr, R. B. (1990). Social support and psychological trauma: A methodological review. *Journal of Traumatic Stress, 3*(4), 593–611. https://doi.org/10.1002/jts.2490030409

Frueh, B. C., Turner, S. M., Beidel, D. C., & Cahill, S. P. (2001). Assessment of social functioning in combat veterans with PTSD. *Aggression and Violent Behavior, 6*(1), 79–90. https://doi.org/10.1016/S1359-1789(99)00012-9

Gelis, A., Cervello, S., Rey, R., Llorca, G., Lambert, P., Franck, N., . . . & Rolland, B. (2020). Peer role-play for training communication skills in medical students: A systematic review. *Simulation in Healthcare, 15*(2), 106–111. https://doi.org/10.1097/SIH.0000000000000412

Gondek, D., Edbrooke-Childs, J., Fink, E., Deighton, J., & Wolpert, M. (2016). Feedback from outcome measures and treatment effectiveness, treatment efficiency, and collaborative practice: A systematic review. *Administration and Policy in Mental Health and Mental Health Services Research, 43*(3), 325–343. https://doi.org/10.1007/s10488-015-0710-5

Goodman, R. (2001). Psychometric properties of the strengths and difficulties questionnaire. *Journal of the American Academy of Child & Adolescent Psychiatry, 40*(11), 1337–1345. https://doi.org/10.1097/00004583-200111000-00015

Greenspan, S. I., DeGangi, G., & Wieder, S. (2001). *The Functional Emotional Assessment Scale (FEAS): For infancy & early childhood*. Interdisciplinary Council on Development & Learning Disorders.

Harmon, C., Hawkins, E. J., Lambert, M. J., Slade, K., & Whipple, J. S. (2005). Improving outcomes for poorly responding clients: The use of clinical support tools and feedback to clients. *Journal of Clinical Psychology, 61*(2), 175–185. https://doi.org/10.1002/jclp.20109

Hayes, S., Strosahl, K., & Wilson, K. (2012). *Acceptance and commitment therapy: The process and practice of mindful change* (2nd ed.). The Guilford Press.

Henrich, S., & Worthington, R. (2021). Let your clients fight dragons: A rapid evidence assessment regarding the therapeutic utility of 'Dungeons & Dragons'. *Journal of Creativity in Mental Health*, 1–19. https://doi.org/10.1080/15401383.2021.1987367

Kashdan, T. B., & Rottenberg, J. (2010). Psychological flexibility as a fundamental aspect of health. *Clinical Psychology Review, 30*(7), 865–878. https://doi.org/10.1016/j.cpr.2010.03.001

Laal, M., Laal, M., & Kermanshahi, Z. K. (2012). 21st century learning; learning in collaboration. *Procedia - Social and Behavioral Sciences, 47*, 1696–1701. https://doi.org/10.1016/j.sbspro.2012.06.885

Laal, M., Naseri, A. S., Laal, M., & Khattami-Kermanshahi, Z. (2013). What do we achieve from learning in collaboration? *Procedia - Social and Behavioral Sciences, 93*, 1427–1432. https://doi.org/10.1016/j.sbspro.2013.10.057

Langberg, J. M., Dvorsky, M. R., & Evans, S. W. (2013). What specific facets of executive function are associated with academic functioning in youth with attention-deficit/hyperactivity disorder? *Journal of Abnormal Child Psychology, 41*(7), 1145–1159. https://doi.org/10.1007/s10802-013-9750-z

Milteer, R. M., Ginsburg, K. R., Council on Communications and Media Committee on Psychosocial Aspects of Child and Family Health, Mulligan, D. A., Ameenuddin, N., Brown, A., . . . & Swanson, W. S. (2012). The importance of play in promoting healthy child development and maintaining strong parent-child bond: Focus on children in poverty. *Pediatrics, 129*(1), e204–e213. https://doi.org/10.1542/peds.2011-2953

Milton, D. E. (2012). On the ontological status of autism: The 'double empathy problem'. *Disability & Society, 27*(6), 883–887. https://doi.org/10.1080/09687599.2012.710008

Mitchell, P., Sheppard, E., & Cassidy, S. (2021). Autism and the double empathy problem: Implications for development and mental health. *British Journal of Developmental Psychology, 39*(1), 1–18. https://doi.org/10.1111/bjdp.12350

Murphy, M., Mathis, E., Weaver, A. D., & Dart, E. (2019). Using antecedent-based strategies to address motivation in behavioral interventions. *Communique, 48*(2), 1–23.

Nakamura, J., & Csikszentmihalyi, M. (2014). The concept of flow. In *Flow and the foundations of positive psychology* (pp. 239–263). Springer.

Nilsen, E. S., & Bacso, S. A. (2017). Cognitive and behavioural predictors of adolescents' communicative perspective-taking and social relationships. *Journal of Adolescence, 56*, 52–63. https://doi.org/10.1016/j.adolescence.2017.01.004

Nilsen, E. S., & Fecica, A. M. (2011). A model of communicative perspective-taking for typical and atypical populations of children. *Developmental Review, 31*(1), 55–78. https://doi.org/10.1016/j.dr.2011.07.001

Percevic, R., Lambert, M. J., & Kordy, H. (2004). Computer-supported monitoring of patient treatment response. *Journal of Clinical Psychology, 60*(3), 285–299. https://doi.org/10.1002/jclp.10264

Pilnick, A., Trusson, D., Beeke, S., O'Brien, R., Goldberg, S., & Harwood, R. H. (2018). Using conversation analysis to inform role play and simulated interaction in communications skills training for healthcare professionals: Identifying avenues for further development through a scoping review. *BMC Medical Education, 18*(1), 1–10. https://doi.org/10.1186/s12909-018-1381-1

Platt, J., Keyes, K. M., & Koenen, K. C. (2014). Size of the social network versus quality of social support: Which is more protective against PTSD? *Social Psychiatry and Psychiatric Epidemiology, 49*(8), 1279–1286. https://doi.org/10.1007/s00127-013-0798-4

Ratcliffe, B., Wong, M., Dossetor, D., & Hayes, S. (2015). The association between social skills and mental health in school-aged children with autism spectrum disorder, with and without intellectual disability. *Journal of Autism and Developmental Disorders, 45*(8), 2487–2496. https://doi.org/10.1007/s10803-015-2411-z

Rubenstein, L. D., Callan, G. L., Ridgley, L. M., & Henderson, A. (2019). Students' strategic planning and strategy use during creative problem solving: The importance of perspective-taking. *Thinking Skills and Creativity, 34*, 100556. https://doi.org/10.1016/j.tsc.2019.02.004

Segrin, C. (2019). Indirect effects of social skills on health through stress and loneliness. *Health Communication, 34*(1), 118–124. https://doi.org/10.1080/10410236.2017.1384434

Segrin, C., McNelis, M., & Swiatkowski, P. (2016). Social skills, social support, and psychological distress: A test of the social skills deficit vulnerability model. *Human Communication Research, 42*(1), 122–137. https://doi.org/10.1111/hcre.12070

Shields, A. M., Cicchetti, D., & Ryan, R. M. (1994). The development of emotional and behavioral self-regulation and social competence among maltreated school-age children. *Development and Psychopathology, 6*(1), 57–75. https://doi.org/10.1017/S0954579400005885

Shimokawa, K., Lambert, M. J., & Smart, D. W. (2010). Enhancing treatment outcome of patients at risk of treatment failure: Meta-analytic and mega-analytic review of a psychotherapy quality assurance system. *Journal of Consulting and Clinical Psychology, 78*(3), 298–311. https://doi.org/10.1037/a0019247

Simoni, Z. R. (2016). Do social skills mediate the relationship between ADHD and depression? *Sociological Spectrum, 36*(2), 109–122. https://doi.org/10.1080/02732173.2015.1095662

Thompson, R. A., & Calkins, S. D. (1996). The double-edged sword: Emotional regulation for children at risk. *Development and Psychopathology, 8*(1), 163–182. https://doi.org/10.1017/S0954579400007021

Todd, A. R., Bodenhausen, G. V., Richeson, J. A., & Galinsky, A. D. (2011). Perspective taking combats automatic expressions of racial bias. *Journal of Personality and Social Psychology, 100*(6), 1027–1042. https://doi.org/10.1037/a0022308

Yee, N., Bailenson, J. N., & Ducheneaut, N. (2009). The Proteus effect: Implications of transformed digital self-representation on online and offline behavior. *Communication Research, 36*(2), 285–312. https://doi.org/10.1177/0093650208330254

Youn, S. J., Kraus, D. R., & Castonguay, L. G. (2012). The treatment outcome package: Facilitating practice and clinically relevant research. *Psychotherapy, 49*(2), 115–122. https://doi.org/10.1037/a0027932

9

Group Development and Therapeutic Factors in Therapeutically Applied Role-Playing Games

The success of therapeutically applied role-playing game (TA-RPG) groups relies on the same theoretical underpinnings as many other group interventions designed for small cohorts. Two of the most popular frameworks for examining group development and value are the stages of group development set forth by Tuckman and Jensen (1977) and the therapeutic factors identified by Yalom (2020). This chapter will discuss the applicability of these understandings as applied to TA-RPGs, as well as encourage facilitators to consider the individual, group, and societal systems present in the treatment context.

Stages of Group Development

The four stages of group development hypothesized by Tuckman in 1965 were "forming," "storming," "norming," and "performing." With a greater understanding of the importance of the termination and end stage of groups, the stage "adjourning" was later added (Tuckman & Jensen, 1977). These stages are believed to apply to any small group of people who work together over time, not just therapeutic or intentional groups. Understanding the five stages of group development is necessary for a TA-RPG facilitator to intentionally support group development.

Forming

In the *forming* stage, the explicit norms of the group are discussed and agreed upon. This can include "session zero" (see Chapter 13) content such as no/please lists, safety tools, and group length, as well as behavioral expectations. The facilitator is the most active and directive during this stage. During gameplay and processing, participants may communicate "through" the facilitator as opposed to directly to each other. Participants new to tabletop role-playing games (TTRPGs) may require more direct instruction of game mechanics and play options.

DOI: 10.4324/9781003281962-9

Storming

In the *storming* stage, participants begin to feel more comfortable disagreeing with one another. There can be a greater presence of notable anxiety and ambiguity as group members test boundaries and start to identify the internal group norms. This is often visible in TTRPG groups when participants and their characters test the boundaries of the game through direct questioning of rules, other characters' actions, or game master (GM) decisions. This may also be visible through player character actions, such as the character engaging in anti-social or disruptive behavior.

Norming

During the *norming* stage, group cohesiveness increases as participants solidify group-specific norms, which decreases ambiguity. These norms can include topics such as how the group responds to participants arriving late or rules regarding sharing personal information. In TA-RPG groups, these norms may be how the group responds to NPCs, if they try to make friends with every creature they find, or how the group responds to violence toward or from one of the player characters.

Performing/Working

The *performing* stage is often referred to as the *working* stage. During this stage, individual and group growth become prevalent, and the group learns to self-regulate. Participants obtain a level of cohesiveness and relationship security to focus their attention on the "work" of the group. This can include addressing individual and group goals. During this stage in a TA-RPG group, participants may make decisions to intentionally support another player's goals. For example, a participant may encourage another participant to speak up during a social encounter to support their previously expressed goal to be more assertive.

Adjourning

The *adjourning* stage is the final phase of the group. During this stage, participants discuss topics related to the graduation of members and/or the group as a whole. Participants explore both progress and loss. Within TA-RPGs, this often takes place during the conclusion of the group's story.

Tuckman's small-group development model is linear, though some theories suggest that group development involves cyclical development through stages (Smith, 2001). Depending on contextual factors and group goals (e.g., deepening relationships, accomplishing an in-game objective) the group's focus and experience may shift between stages.

This cyclical pattern can be observed in TA-RPG groups. For example, a group may exist in the working stage when overcoming a challenge in an adventure, but through the course of that challenge identify an interpersonal conflict or difference in priorities that will push the group back into a storming stage. This cyclical nature of development should not be seen as a setback. It is likely that the group's previous experiences with storming, norming, and performing set them up to engage in the next cycle of storming with increased complexity and success.

Group Development in Cohort and Rolling Admission Groups

Some groups are "cohort groups," in which the group members all join at the same time. Cohort group members are all on the same level of newness in the group though they may have varying experiences in regard to therapy groups and TTRPGs. Rolling admission groups, in contrast, support participants entering the group at staggered intervals, with new group members joining as existing group members leave (through graduation or early termination). Cohort groups move through the stages of group development together. In contrast, rolling admission groups may experience micro and macro levels of group development. The micro level of group development refers to the group members who are currently present in the group, and it may at any time consist of participants who have been in the group for long periods, as well as those who are brand new to the group. Over time, the current group members will strengthen cohesion, increase their comfort with healthy conflict, and develop norms of working and playing together.

This micro development may be supported by the macro group development. The macro group development refers to the development of norms and expectations of the group, above and beyond that extend past its current members. Implicit and explicit norms developed by previous group members are likely to be carried forward through new members such that the norms may continue to exist even though none of the original members who established those norms are still participating. For example, in a six-month-old group, newer members may observe established group members share personal connections between in-game experiences and real-life experiences, and then engage in the modeled behaviors themselves without prompting. Additionally, established group members may provide explicit instructions about group norms, demonstrate trust in the facilitator and group process, and share personal stories of growth stemming from participation in the group to new members. The imparting of such information may hasten the comfort of new members and support the installation of hope (Yalom &

Leszcz, 2020). At this time, further research into the development of TA-RPG groups in cohort and rolling admission remains warranted.

Therapeutic Factors in Group Interventions

Irvin Yalom, a predominant scholar in the effectiveness and utility of group therapy interventions, identified 11 primary therapeutic factors in group therapy (Yalom & Leszcz, 2020). Since the identification of these factors, they have been used as a framework through which to understand functions of group interventions and factors impacting change. These factors are not considered to be wholly distinct; instead, there is an expectation of overlap between the factors. Further, these factors are considered to be interdependent in both appearance and function (Yalom & Leszcz, 2020). The salience of each therapeutic factor will vary based on the type of group, the needs of the participants, and the developmental stage of the group. Additionally, though many aspects of these therapeutic factors occur spontaneously and without conscious intent throughout the group, some aspects require the support of intentional cultivation and development by the facilitator. The way in which each of these therapeutic factors manifest in a group can vary due to group type and participant presentation and needs. Though group interventions work with multiple participants at a time, each individual in a group may have their own distinct goals and needs. Further, the factors discussed in the following were originally conceived from a Western perspective and designed for use within a Western societal and treatment context. Facilitators should be mindful to evaluate the use and prioritization of these factors through the lenses most relevant to each group's participants.

Therapeutic Factors:

- Instillation of Hope
- Universality
- Imparting of Information
- Altruism
- Corrective Recapitulation
- Development of Social Skills
- Imitative Behavior
- Interpersonal Learning
- Group Cohesiveness
- Catharsis
- Existential Factors

Instillation of Hope

Research has consistently found a strong positive correlation between successful treatment outcomes and participant's hope that treatment will be helpful (Bartholomew et al., 2021; Irving et al., 2004; Gilman et al., 2012). Hope that one will benefit from treatment can support increased engagement in therapy, supporting a self-fulfilling prophecy where increased engagement and adherence to treatment support positive outcomes. Consistent with the common factor of treatment expectations (discussed in Chapter 13), when participant and facilitator are aligned in their expectations, achievements of those expectations are more likely (Seligman, 1995). Participation in group treatment allows group members to observe and learn from others in treatment with similar identities or challenges, but may be at a different point in the change process. This allows participants to gather information about efficacy of treatment expectations not only from their own experiences and the facilitator, but from their peers in the group as well (Yalom & Leszcz, 2020).

TA-RPG groups support installation of hope through several mechanisms. The novelty of the TA-RPG group format is unlikely to "feel" like a typical therapy group to most participants. Additionally, participants have the opportunity to actively participate in the group without the expectation of immediately sharing details about their background or inner experience. Further, group members often experience the benefits of group participation early on, such as through gaining insight into the ways in which one's character acts like themselves. An example comes from a TA-RPG group for veterans diagnosed with posttraumatic stress disorder (PTSD). During the first session, the potential of this group was noted by one of the participants. The facilitator introduced a classic tavern scene and invited participants to place miniatures representing their character on a map, then describe what their character was doing within the busy tavern. Participants placed their characters around the walls of the tavern and described engaging in vigilance-related tasks—scanning the area, listening for unexpected noises, assessing patrons for potential threats. The last participant to place their character on the map leaned back in his chair, examined the map for a moment, and expressed "Well, [shoot]. I just noticed we placed all our characters with their backs to the wall, scanning the surroundings like we do in real life. This is us. I can see how this is going to be helpful."

Universality

Group therapy creates opportunities for participants to interact with others with similar experiences and can help participants realize they are not alone in their problems (Yalom & Leszcz, 2020). Many individuals, especially those who have been minoritized (e.g., due to identity or experience), hold thoughts or beliefs that they are uniquely broken, unlovable, or unacceptable. These beliefs can be further exacerbated by social isolation. Group interventions create opportunities to more accurately observe the experiences of peers aside from the glimpses they may see on social media. Groups that are offered for those who hold a shared identity, such as LGBTQIA+ groups, neurodivergent groups, or groups for individuals who have experienced trauma, have a clear starting point from which to identify areas of universality. Even in groups that have more open-ended participation requirements, identifying shared areas of vulnerability and connection can be a powerful tool to support connection between participants and challenge beliefs related to isolation (Yalom & Leszcz, 2020).

TA-RPGs may be uniquely suited to further support the experience of universality through narrative and gameplay opportunities (e.g., interacting with non-player characters (NPCs)). In the game, an NPC might ask explicit questions about a particular struggle: "I have been feeling really down lately, and it's getting in the way of my magical abilities. I feel so useless. Have any of y'all felt this way before?" Alternatively, the NPC could make statements with a more implicit ask: "I feel so down and useless lately. I don't think I can help you on your quest while I feel this way." Both of these statements can serve to normalize struggles with mood, and create opportunities for participants to discuss their experiences through their character.

A Tale From the Real-World Table

In a TA-RPG group of military veterans, several of the participants had expressed challenges related to impulsivity and hypervigilance. In the game, the group was traveling down a road through a forest, following the trail of several bandits who had kidnapped two village children. The players had described themselves as alert to any threat, and were actively scanning the environment for potential threats. While moving down the road, the party heard a rustling noise in the bushes to their right, and all of a sudden, a small figure leaped out of the bush. "I stab it with my knife!" exclaimed the lead party member, before the facilitator was able to explain that what jumped out of the bushes was an adorable, small creature resembling a bear cub, covered in feathers with a short beak where a bear's snout would be. In this moment, the facilitator had several options—they could ask the participant to hold their reaction until the description was finished to allow the participant to re-think their action, they could ask the participant to roll a "perception check" to see if their character was able to get a clear view of the creature before attempting to stab it, or they could ask the participant to roll an attack to see if the character was able to stab the small creature. The facilitator made the decision to ask for an attack roll, consistent with the participant's initial declaration, as well as their expressed difficulties with impulse control and frustration tolerance. The attempt to stab the creature was successful, resulting in its death. All the players reacted with distress when they realized the character stabbed a small defenseless creature, as they were faced with the manifestation of hypervigilant reactivity. During the processing portion of the group, the player whose character attacked the creature expressed shame and guilt, before relating the experience to other moments in his life. He expressed that though he does not physically hurt people in real life, his hypervigilance and reactions to perceived threats often led to problems at work, as well as in relationships with friends, family, and medical providers. The participant further disclosed that these experiences led him to believe that he is a bad person. Other group members were quick to jump in with similar experiences and fears. The group members expressed an appreciation that the game format allowed them to see the process "play out" in a way they were unable to see in their daily lives. Additionally, though they noted this experience did not eliminate the shame many of them felt in response to the hypervigilance reaction patterns in their lives, several expressed appreciation at the realization they were not alone in these struggles.

Imparting of Information

Imparting of information includes the direct sharing of informal information or guidance to participants from peers or the facilitator, as well as direct formal instruction from facilitators (Yalom & Leszcz, 2020). Much of the educational aspects of group therapy and TA-RPGs are implicit; however, there are times in which explicitly teaching skills or giving advice occurs. When this explicit instruction happens, an atmosphere of collaborative participation is key in order to avoid participants feeling patronized (Yalom & Leszcz, 2020).

Imparting of information begins during the screening process, where participants should be provided information about what to expect in the group and have opportunities to ask questions about group processes and norms. Once the group has begun, direct imparting of information from facilitator to participants and participant to participant is often more common at the beginning of a group, as members are learning how to relate to each other, the facilitator, and the game. Participants may have questions about the game or offer guidance to other participants who are less familiar with TTRPGs. Advice giving between participants can be considered as a way participants attempt to manage their relationships with each other (Yalom & Leszcz, 2020). When participants give advice to other participants, they take on the less emotionally vulnerable role of "helper." That being said, advice giving from one participant to another typically demonstrates caring and engagement. If the facilitator effectively uses functional analysis in these advice-giving scenarios, they may be able to identify what the participant is trying to accomplish with their helping behavior and support the participant's development of interpersonal connection skills.

When the facilitator has explicit guidance or instruction to offer the group, they can utilize in-game NPCs as a way of providing such information within the narrative framework, shifting the role of "teacher" from the facilitator to an in-game character. Such a shift allows for covert didactic communication, which can serve as a more approachable method of instruction for some participants. Facilitators may create an NPC who is a mentor to the group, providing direct instruction about what the group should do next or handle a particular problem. The facilitator may choose to exaggerate the mentor character and make them hilariously long-winded, patronizing, or boring, as a way to introduce levity and engagement into what could otherwise be a boring and didactic encounter reminiscent of a particularly dry day at school. Alternatively, the so-called mentor could be more of the bumbling variety—needing the group's support and help more than providing answers to the group. This type of companion could support the group through the Socratic model, asking questions until participants reach the answers they seek. Narrative gameplay creates opportunities for learning through interactions with a multitude of different NPCs—if the group does not find a particular method engaging, the facilitator is encouraged to shift to a different NPC or tactic altogether, without breaking narrative immersion.

Altruism

Many group therapy participants enter treatment with low self-esteem and a fear or expectation that they have little to offer others (Yalom & Leszcz, 2020). Through participation in TA-RPGs, they have the opportunity to offer support to other participants around the table. The opportunity to help others and be successful in these encounters can support participants' sense of self-efficacy and build self-esteem.

Many TA-RPG storylines feature multiple opportunities to rescue NPCs, and lift the lives of towns, countries, even whole worlds! Characters in TTRPGs are often set up to be the heroes of the story—and these narratives can invite opportunities for good deeds between characters and NPCs. The adventuring party may take on a quest to save a struggling magical creature, protect a town from invasion, or discover an infinite source of power from deep within a cave. The opportunities for altruism can be broad, adventure-long goals, or worked into the fabric of singular encounters. Encounter-level opportunities for altruism include standing up for an NPC in a conflict, casting a support spell on a fellow character during a battle, or rescuing a kitten from a tree.

At times, group members may rebuff in-game offers of altruism from other participants. This may be related to mistrust of the other participant's intentions, a misunderstanding of the situation, or a belief that they do not deserve to be the recipient of such altruism. When such attempts at altruism occur within the context of the game, playing this out at the character level can allow the facilitator (or the facilitator's NPCs) to ask questions of the participant about their character's understanding and intentions. Using the character, instead of the participant, extends the aesthetic distance between the participant and their character, allowing the participant to place their fears or concerns on their character and talk about their concerns more readily.

Corrective Recapitulation

Often identified as "Corrective Recapitulation of the Primary Family Group," this factor refers to the phenomenon within therapy groups to recreate common challenging interpersonal dynamics experienced in the participant's original family group, but with the opportunity to resolve the new instances of such dynamics in more rewarding and adaptive ways (Yalom & Leszcz, 2020). This concept has since been applied to maladaptive interpersonal patterns more broadly than just those from an original family makeup, with similar opportunities for corrective experiences in the group (Bieling, 2009). This factor rests on the understanding that when a participant joins a group, they bring with them all their previously established ways of relating to and understanding the world. Within the context of the group, participants are expected to elicit the same particular behaviors from others and react with the same established patterns of behavior to particular situations that they would within their everyday lives outside of the group. However, unlike everyday life, participants in therapy groups have the support of the facilitator and the intention and willingness of the other participants to support positive interpersonal outcomes. In TA-RPG groups in particular, these interactions are often played out through character relationships. The extra space and opportunities to suspend or slow time as needed create added opportunities for identifying and trying out new styles of reacting.

When maladaptive relational patterns are identified within a group, it is important to provide opportunities for change and corrective experiences.

If a participant's negative expectations, especially those related to rejection, failure, or neglect, are reinforced in a TA-RPG group, their experience of safety within the group can be diminished, further entrenching the pattern of expectation. For example, many participants engage in self-protective behavior designed to elicit rejection from peers, wherein they errantly perceive their own rejection to be inevitable and behave in ways that are designed to hasten that outcome. When this behavior is identified by the facilitator, they should respond in such a way that makes it clear to the participant that the participant will not be rejected, despite inappropriate behavior on their part or the part of their character.

Development of Social Skills

The development of interpersonal skills occurs in every therapy group to varying extents; however, the specific skills and type of instruction vary between groups based on group type and participant needs (Yalom & Leszcz, 2020). The development of social skills in the context of peer groups can be especially valuable, as it provides opportunities for behavioral rehearsal and feedback between participants. Feedback is often pertinent to environments beyond the therapy room, especially for adolescents who seek out and value feedback from their peers above that which they receive from adults (Bednar & Fisher, 2003). The development of effective feedback strategies can be especially beneficial for clients working to reduce miscommunication in their relationships. In therapy groups, participants can have the opportunity to learn when their intended message does not line up with the message received by the listener (Leszcz & Malat, 2011).

TA-RPGs are well suited to support the development of social skills through both explicit and implicit experiential learning. Participants have opportunities to participate in safe socialization with peers both around the game table and within the game. Though it is unlikely participants will need to convince the queen of an invading zombie hoard in real life, a participant has the opportunity to practice persuasion and self-advocacy skills while being encouraged by their peers and scaffolded by the facilitator. TA-RPG groups use the same rationale of role-play employed by many other therapy groups, with an added layer of interest, engagement, and flexibility often notably lacking from scripted or contrived role-play exercises.

Imitative Behavior

During TA-RPG groups, participants have the option to observe and replicate behaviors modeled by their peers, NPCs, and the facilitator. There is strong evidence that facilitators can support adaptive communication patterns in groups by modeling appropriate self-disclosure, compassionate feedback, and support (Bernard et al., 2008). Similarly, group members are presented opportunities to observe peers who have mastered certain skills, as well as peers who are in the process of developing mastery of new skills.

Imitative behavior typically manifests early on in a group's life cycle, when participants are using the facilitator or more experienced members as models for effective in-group behavior (Colijn, 1991). Facilitators can utilize NPCs within the game to further model adaptive behavior or to create opportunities for participants to follow an NPC's lead as a way to encourage novel action among players who may be anxious or uncertain about how to proceed. Additionally, facilitators can create in-game opportunities for players to model a skill or talent. For example, an NPC aligned with the party could take the lead on a tricky conversation or take the first step of brainstorming ideas to get into a locked room.

A Tale From the Real-World Table

When Sam started in the group, they had limited knowledge about TTRPGs, waited for the opinions of the rest of the group before weighing in, and would only participate in stressful social encounters with other characters present. Sam's treatment goals included increased comfort and frequency of role-playing their character, Skyre, as well as increased confidence around spontaneous or stressful communication. The facilitator had been observing regular gains related to these goals. In the storyline, the adventuring party was attempting to send a few of their members to investigate an underground organization that was trying to take over the world with giant zombie starfish. To accomplish this task, the characters opted to undergo a job interview to infiltrate the ranks of this nefarious organization. The facilitator specifically aligned the job requirements with Skyre's skills so they would feel more comfortable volunteering. Sam used Skyre to step up to the job, imitating communication skills observed from fellow participants, NPCs, and the facilitator. During the interview process, Skyre gave a rousing speech, enacted by Sam, about how they were the best fit for the job. They confidently answered several "tricky" questions, and the interviewer (played by the facilitator) was immensely impressed. Following this performance, several group members praised and reinforced Sam's performance of Skyre, noting both their interview prowess and their calm during a stressful process.

Interpersonal Learning

Interpersonal learning is an excellent example of the ways in which the therapeutic factors co-occur and co-mingle. Interpersonal learning relies on an understanding of the function of interpersonal relationships in health and personal growth, the power of corrective emotional experiences, and the existence of the group as a social microcosm (Yalom & Leszcz, 2020). The study of interpersonal relationships and attachment supports the idea that individuals exist within a relational matrix, best understood within the context of our current and past relationships (Waldinger & Schulz, 2016). Further, social isolation and loneliness is a risk factor for early mortality (Holt-Lunstad et al., 2010). Peer, parental, and teacher support have all been shown to be protective factors that reduce negative outcomes related to peer victimization in preadolescence and adolescence (McDougall & Vaillancourt, 2015). In therapy groups, participants have opportunities to learn from each other through direct feedback, collaboration, and observation. Participants who do not yet feel comfortable discussing problems or insecurities with the group can still benefit from seeing similar problems tackled by peers, often referred to as vicarious therapy (Moreno, 1939).

TA-RPG groups provide a multitude of pathways for interpersonal learning. Player characters and NPCs create opportunities for learning to occur between group members around the table, as well as in the game through their in-game avatars. Additionally, the facilitator can design and utilize NPCs with specific interaction styles to support participant learning. For example, in a group where the participants struggled to listen to each other, the facilitator could introduce an NPC who interrupted all the players to an exaggerated degree. If executed with the appropriate levity, this could create opportunities for the players to build insight into the way that interrupting impacts them and their peers, and collaborate on solutions to the problem. The group can then practice giving feedback, setting boundaries, and coaching with this NPC. Alternatively, in the same group, the facilitator may introduce an NPC that will not tolerate interruptions and who hates when people talk over each other. In this scenario, the adventuring party may need to access information this NPC has, but refuses to pass on, unless the group can stop speaking over each other. Utilizing either of these NPC scenarios allows the facilitator to interact with the players through the medium of a character, which provides the facilitator more flexibility in interaction styles than if they were acting as themselves.

Group Cohesiveness

Group cohesiveness refers to how connected the group members are to each other, to the group as a whole, and to the group's goals. This can be seen as the group corollary to working alliance in individual psychotherapy, the active and cooperative relationship between client and therapist (Yalom & Leszcz, 2020). Consistent with individual therapy, the group relationship, or cohesiveness, is a strong predictor of outcome in therapy groups (Burlingame et al., 2018; Marmarosh et al., 2005; Marmarosh & Sproul, 2021).

In TA-RPG groups, participants are provided opportunities through the narrative of the game to work together toward a common goal. TTRPGs are inherently cooperative, with the group set up to work together to complete a mission—whether that is uncovering a lost relic, defeating a great evil, or starting a successful magical cruise line. Furthermore, facilitators can manipulate the storyline and environment to support the development of group cohesion. The facilitator may adjust encounters to rely on the skills of multiple characters in concert, or adjust the constraints of the environment to keep party members together to promote opportunities for communication.

A Tale From the Real-World Table

An established TA-RPG group of adolescent girls were in search of the three pieces of a magical staff that would give them the power needed to quell a dragon that had been terrorizing a nearby village. The adventuring party had traveled deep into abandoned mines in search of the three pieces, rumored to all be stored somewhere in the mines. During previous sessions, some disagreements about strategies and tactics had arisen, but were quickly dismissed by the players before they could be resolved. In the mines, when disagreements about tactics again arose, participants decided to split the party (ostensibly to avoid conflict). The party split-up, struggling to complete their mission until they found a magical divining rod and learned the three pieces had been magically concealed, unable to be detected without the aid of the divining rod. The rod was introduced by the facilitator as a narrative means of incentivizing the characters (and by proxy, the players) to explore together. The players identified the benefit of staying near each other, even though this created more opportunities for tension and conflict. Although the players quickly uncovered the first piece, disagreements continued while looking for the next component. However, in context of their recent success, and with the knowledge they would need to stick together to find the next component, the players were now uniquely motivated to re-engage with and resolve their conflict instead of engaging in continued avoidance. The facilitator scaffolded the participant's engagement in conflict resolution by asking questions about intent, and created opportunities for continued collaboration and success through small environmental challenges that required the support of multiple party members to successfully navigate (i.e., locked doors that required multiple buttons, yards apart, to be depressed at the same time to open).

Catharsis

Catharsis is an emotional release, often where participants display their unfiltered or raw emotions. This can be an important part of building insight and the healing process, but it is important to note that catharsis alone is not sufficient to predict positive change (Yalom & Leszcz, 2020). In the context of group therapy, catharsis is considered part of the process of learning to engage in effective emotional disclosure. Cathartic events can be remarkable and memorable in therapy, and are often cited by group therapy participants as significant events in treatment (Ahmed et al., 2010). An example of this assertion comes from a study of adolescent girls in therapy that utilized expressive arts (e.g., guided drawing, painting, and writing exercises) as part of group therapy. In this study, they found that catharsis was highly linked to measured therapeutic alliance—participants may have felt sufficiently safe to express themselves and develop trust following moments when their raw expressions of emotion did not lead to rejection from the group (Adibah & Zakaria, 2015).

Catharsis is an excellent example of the interconnectedness of the therapeutic factors—catharsis alone is unlikely to spark meaningful change without insight. Such insight may not be possible without cohesion within the group and opportunities for interpersonal learning. TA-RPGs can provide space for participants to experience catharsis in a safe and low-stakes way through their characters in the fantasy space. Participants also have the opportunity to reflect on the actions of their character—to identify what worked and what did not about their character's emotional expression. Because the focus can be on the *character's* actions instead of the player's, participants may experience less guilt or shame around such displays of emotion. The facilitator can support the player by engaging through a lens of acceptance and curiosity, supporting the player by inquiring what led to the emotions and the outburst. Over time, participants can gain practice noticing and expressing their emotions as they come up. Allowing for opportunities of catharsis through one's character can decrease fears surrounding vulnerability while increasing a player's ability to regulate their emotions.

Existential Factors

Existential factors refers to a collection of sentiments related to the presumed "human condition" (Yalom & Leszcz, 2020). The existential factors are deeply tied to concepts such as purpose, free will, responsibility, sentience, and values. This collection includes the understanding that life is not always fair or just, that one cannot escape from all pain or death, that even if one has support and direction from others they ultimately have responsibility for the decisions they make, and that meaning is not innately imbued on any one individual. A focus on existential factors is common in groups designed to address specific topics related to illness, death, and substance use (Yalom & Leszcz, 2020). Members of these specific topic groups may find that the events that contributed to their increased awareness around mortality and individual responsibility had the beneficial effect of helping them identify and more closely align with their values (Antoni et al., 2001).

The purpose of existential factors is not to increase avoidance and depression in participants. Indeed, the opposite is true. Fear around death, loneliness, and failure often prevent participants from engaging in valued activities. Normalizing and naming their fears can help participants acknowledge these barriers and make intentional decisions related to their personal values.

Though the degree to which existential factors are explicitly introduced in TA-RPG groups varies by group goals, populations, and intentions, many of these concepts will be addressed implicitly through the narrative of the game. Participants have the opportunity to explore and construct meaning within the worlds they help to create. When appropriate, character retirement or death can act as a corollary to their own mortality. Throughout the story, group members have opportunities to solicit feedback about what their character should do, but ultimately get to make their own decisions for their character's actions and reactions. Even if the civilizations depicted in a group's story are a utopia (they often are not), the roll of the dice creates opportunities to respond to randomness and luck (or lack thereof). Finally, players can explore their own values and purpose through their character. Though characters may be set up to fulfill a certain role in a story (i.e., the heroes), players get to determine how their characters fulfill that role, if at all.

Systems in the Room

When working with TA-RPG groups, similar to any other therapeutic intervention, it is important to consider the context of the group and individuals that comprise it. Loosely building off the bioecological model, we identify several areas of personal identity, as well as group, family, and societal contexts to which the facilitator of a TA-RPG group should be mindful (Bronfenbrenner & Ceci, 1994; Bronfenbrenner & Morris, 2005). Each of these areas should be viewed in relation to the other areas, as the intersectionality of these systems cannot be ignored. For example, a 12-year-old participant in a group of other 12-year-olds will have a different experience than a 12-year-old in a group of 16-year-olds, due to the group makeup in relation to their age. Understanding the systems within which a participant exists will help facilitators to conceptualize cases for treatment planning purposes, identify appropriate group makeup, develop group-appropriate storylines, and utilize facilitation strategies most appropriate to the participant.

Individual

Individual factors are any factors directly related to a participant's history, experience, preferences, identity, strengths, and challenges. This can include the participant's play style or knowledge of TTRPGs, comfort level with sharing emotions, interpersonal skills, and goals for therapy. Individual factors also include demographic or diversity characteristics, including age, gender, medical or psychiatric diagnoses, race, and economic status. Furthermore, this category includes situational or transient factors, such as sleep, stressful internal events, and acute injuries. Some of these factors are heavily influenced by society and/or the participant's history of experience with these factors (e.g., a participant who has been told they are "bad" at math may develop a lower frustration tolerance to math-related activities). The facilitator's awareness of individual factors can help them to identify appropriate group placement for participants, as well as to support their use of functional analysis during group sessions. For instance, if a participant seems disinterested in using their most powerful attack in combat (which requires adding up the results of multiple dice), and the facilitator is aware they have challenges with math, the facilitator may hypothesize that anxiety around math is contributing to this behavior.

Group

Group factors include the makeup of the group's participants, the group's needs, goals, and the level of group cohesion. Further, group factors reflect each participant's individual factors and how those interact with each other in a group space. Understanding the make-up of the group is necessary for the facilitator to set appropriate goals, support the development of group norms, and create an effective learning environment for the participants. To illustrate this, consider a group of participants who demonstrate rapid processing speeds in their cognition and rapid response time in their communication. If another participant needs five to ten seconds after hearing a prompt to process and respond (individual factor), the facilitator should be intentional about creating participation structures or norms around communication that support each participant's ability to communicate.

Setting

The setting of the group can greatly influence participants' needs, methods for increasing engagement, and even the appropriateness of certain safety tools. For example, groups delivered virtually eliminate the need for transportation to and from a physical location. As such, they may be a great fit for individuals who have mobility challenges, need regular access to hard-to-transport medical equipment, or have limited access to reliable transportation. However, they require a quiet space, strong Internet connection, and a video/microphone set-up. When determining the right setting for a group, the facilitator should consider the access needs of the participants, as well as the feasibility of the options for the facilitator.

Communities

The communities to which a participant belongs will influence the participant's interests, beliefs, and interpersonal capacities. For the purposes of TA-RPGs, "communities" refer to family groups, religious communities, sport/academic/extracurricular groups, and other formal and informal organizations the participant is involved in. The facilitator's awareness of the communities a participant is in can support the facilitator in meeting a participant's logistic needs (e.g., not scheduling a group on a religious holiday), in designing narratives to fit a participant's interests, as well as in awareness of environmental stressors. If a participant belongs to a community that is experiencing discrimination, a facilitator's awareness of both individual and community factors can support the facilitator in developing narratives that best support the participant's experience based on the participant's goals and preferences.

Society

Societal factors include the moral and religious belief systems within larger society groups, systems of privilege and oppression, and important society-impacting events. An understanding and acknowledgment of these systems can help the facilitator to create a safe space for participants. As with any of these systems, the facilitator should be aware of changes in these systems and respond accordingly when appropriate. As an example, when the COVID-19 pandemic began sweeping through the United States in 2020, one of the authors was running a TA-RPG group with a storyline where the adventuring party was attempting to stop a magical sickness that was sweeping the land. The facilitator was aware of the real-life corollary, and with the participant's approval, they quickly resolved the storyline and shifted the narrative focus to an alternative story. This successful shift was reliant on the facilitator's knowledge of this societal factor and its likely impact on participants, as well as their knowledge of the group's preferences, goals, and norms around communication.

References

Adibah, S. M., & Zakaria, M. (2015). The efficacy of expressive arts therapy in the creation of catharsis in counseling. *Mediterranean Journal of Social Sciences, 6*(6 S1), 298. https://doi.org/10.5901/mjss.2015.v6n6s1p298

Ahmed, S., Abolmagd, S., Rakhawy, M., Erfan, S., & Mamdouh, R. (2010). Therapeutic factors in group psychotherapy: A study of Egyptian drug addicts. *Journal of Groups in Addiction & Recovery, 5*(3–4), 194–213. https://doi.org/10.1080/1556035X.2010.523345

Antoni, M. H., Lehman, J. M., Kilbourn, K. M., Boyers, A. E., Culver, J. L., Alferi, S. M., . . . & Carver, C. S. (2001). Cognitive-behavioral stress management intervention decreases the prevalence of depression and enhances benefit finding among women under treatment for early-stage breast cancer. *Health Psychology, 20*(1), 20–32. https://doi.org/10.1037/0278-6133.20.1.20

Bartholomew, T. T., Joy, E. E., & Gundel, B. E. (2021). Clients' hope for counseling as a predictor of outcome in psychotherapy. *The Counseling Psychologist, 49*(8), 1126–1146.

Bednar, D. E., & Fisher, T. D. (2003). Peer referencing in adolescent decision making as a function of perceived parenting style. *Adolescence, 38*(152). Retrieved on June 13, 2022, from https://europepmc.org/article/med/15053489.

Bernard, H., Burlingame, G., Flores, P., Greene, L., Joyce, A., Kobos, J. C., . . . & Feirman, D. (2008). Clinical practice guidelines for group psychotherapy. *International Journal of Group Psychotherapy, 58*(4), 455–542. https://doi.org/10.1521/ijgp.2008.58.4.455

Bieling, P. J., McCabe, R. E., & Antony, M. M. (2009). *Cognitive-behavioral therapy in groups.* Guilford Press.

Bronfenbrenner, U., & Ceci, S. J. (1994). Nature-nurture reconceptualized in developmental perspective: A bioecological model. *Psychological Review, 101*(4), 568–586.

Bronfenbrenner, U., & Morris P. A. (2005). The bioecological model of human development. In W. Damon, R. M. Lerner & R. M. Lerner (Eds.), *Handbook of child psychology.* Wiley. https://doi.org/10.1002/9780470147658.chpsy0114

Burlingame, G. M., McClendon, D. T., & Yang, C. (2018). Cohesion in group therapy: A meta-analysis. *Psychotherapy, 55*(4), 384–398. https://doi.org/10.1037/pst0000173

Colijn, S., Hoencamp, E., Snijders, H. J., van der Spek, M. W., & Duivenvoorden, H. J. (1991). A comparison of curative factors in different types of group psychotherapy. *International Journal of Group Psychotherapy, 41*(3), 365–378.

Gilman, R., Schumm, J. A., & Chard, K. M. (2012). Hope as a change mechanism in the treatment of posttraumatic stress disorder. *Psychological Trauma: Theory, Research, Practice, and Policy, 4*(3), 270–277. https://doi.org/10.1037/a0024252

Holt-Lunstad, J., Smith, T. B., & Layton, J. B. (2010). Social relationships and mortality risk: A meta-analytic review. *PLoS Medicine, 7*(7). https://doi.org/10.1371/journal.pmed.1000316

Irving, L. M., Snyder, C. R., Cheavens, J., Gravel, L., Hanke, J., Hilberg, P., & Nelson, N. (2004). The relationships between hope and outcomes at the pretreatment, beginning, and later phases of psychotherapy. *Journal of Psychotherapy Integration, 14*(4), 419–443. https://doi.org/10.1037/1053-0479.14.4.419

Leszcz, M., & Malat, J. (2011). The interpersonal model of group psychotherapy. In J. Kleinberg (Ed.), *The Wiley-Blackwell handbook of group psychotherapy* (pp. 33–58). John Wiley & Sons, Ltd. https://doi.org/10.1002/9781119950882

Marmarosh, C., Holtz, A., & Schottenbauer, M. (2005). Group cohesiveness, group-derived collective self-esteem, group-derived hope, and the well-being of group therapy members. *Group Dynamics: Theory, Research, and Practice, 9*(1), 32–44. https://doi.org/10.1037/1089-2699.9.1.32

Marmarosh, C. L., & Sproul, A. (2021). Group cohesion: Empirical evidence from group psychotherapy for those studying other areas of group work. In C. D. Parks & G. A. Tasca (Eds.), *The psychology of groups: The intersection of social psychology and psychotherapy research* (pp. 169–189). American Psychological Association. https://doi.org/10.1037/0000201-010

McDougall, P., & Vaillancourt, T. (2015). Long-term adult outcomes of peer victimization in childhood and adolescence: Pathways to adjustment and maladjustment. *American Psychologist, 70*(4), 300–310. https://doi.org/10.1037/a0039174

Moreno, J. L. (1939). Psychodramatic shock therapy: A sociometric approach to the problem of mental disorders. *Sociometry, 2,* 1–30.

Seligman, M. E. P. (1995). The effectiveness of psychotherapy: The Consumer Reports study. *American Psychologist, 50*(12), 965–974. https://doi.org/10.1037/0003-066X.50.12.965

Smith, G. (2001). Group development: A review of the literature and a commentary on future research directions. *Group Facilitation, 3*(Spring), 14–45.

Tuckman, B. W., & Jensen, M. A. C. (1977). Stages of small-group development revisited. *Group & Organization Studies, 2*(4), 419–427. https://doi.org/10.1177/105960117700200404

Waldinger, R. J., & Schulz, M. S. (2016). The long reach of nurturing family environments: Links with midlife emotion-regulatory styles and late-life security in intimate relationships. *Psychological Science, 27*(11), 1443–1450. https://doi.org/10.1177/0956797616661556

Yalom, I., & Leszcz, M. (2020). *Theory and practice of group psychotherapy* (6th ed.). Basic Books.

10

Session Design in the Game to Grow Method of Therapeutically Applied Role-Playing Games

While therapeutically applied role-playing games (TA-RPGs) may appear as simply a fun and engaging relational play experience on the surface, similar to a recreational tabletop role-playing game (TTRPG) play, in TA-RPGs the therapeutic game master (GM) will suffuse intentional, therapeutically relevant material throughout the experience. TA-RPG facilitators build participation structures into their pre- and post-gameplay content that will encourage engagement, support reflection, and catalyze insight. Using the DOTS System of Narrative Construction, therapeutic GMs will design gameplay content in alignment with treatment goals. This tool supports the foundational narrative structure of the gameplay experience and provides multiple access points to incorporate therapeutic content directly into the narrative.

Session Layout

A Game to Grow TA-RPG session is arranged in the following structure:

- Check-In
- Story Recap
- Gameplay
- Check-Out
- Group Processing (if a counseling group)

A key difference between counseling TA-RPG groups and social flourishing TA-RPG groups designed to provide social support and build social confidence is the session structure. Counseling TA-RPG groups are 120 minutes long, with five minutes for check-in, 80 minutes for gameplay, 30 minutes for processing, and five minutes for check-out.

Social Flourishing groups are typically 90 minutes in length, with ten minutes dedicated to the check-in process, 75 minutes for game-play, and 5 minutes for the check-out process.

DOI: 10.4324/9781003281962-10

Though the duration of groups should be adjusted to fit the setting, the proportions of the session allocated to various processes should be roughly as outlined in the following and maintained with consistency. Experienced TTRPG players may note that these times are significantly shorter than many social TTRPG group durations (often four to six hours of gameplay). This is an intentional choice to support the goals for the group. To keep engagement high, TA-RPG groups must not meet for longer than participants' general stamina will last. Ending the gameplay while the participants are still enjoying the activity leaves them eager to return when the session ends. This continuation desire supports consistent participant attendance. Additionally, groups should not attempt to create opportunities for too much learning without adequate space to reflect and internalize the growth. Shorter sessions (i.e., on a weekly basis) allow for a learning structure that supports continued engagement and provide frequent opportunities for participants to regularly connect in-game experiences to their lived experience.

Check-In

For many group participants, engaging in loosely structured narrative social play will be challenging, especially if they are struggling with social anxiety or have not had a history of rewarding social experiences. The check-in process, a structured social experience with clearly defined and outlined participation structures, provides a warm-up to the social engagement of the gameplay portion of the session.

Check-In Questions

Check-in questions are leveraged to orient group members, elicit interpersonal communication, inspire players to create details about their character's past and inner world, and prompt players to compare and contrast their own experience with their character's experience. Check-in questions may be as simple as "What is a piece of art you enjoy?" or "What is your favorite food?" when the group is first forming. Once group rapport has been established, check-in questions may require more reflection and vulnerability such as "What is something you look for in a friend?" or "What is a strength you and your character share?" These questions provide a structured opportunity for each participant to share something about themselves with the group, experience being witnessed and honored in their sharing, and provide the same honor to their group members. The group facilitator should also answer the check-in question, as it provides an opportunity for modeling and increased rapport building.

For an in-game bonus, clients are offered an optional follow-up question, often creating an opportunity to expand on their answer or to answer for or as their character. Answering as their character creates an opportunity for the participant to practice speaking as their character in the first person. Participants may be invited to alter their voice and mannerisms, or simply use the first-person language. The in-game bonus for the follow-up question is typically a token they can redeem to allow *another* player to re-roll dice when the outcome of a dice roll was unfavorable. As always, this tool should be adjusted to specific populations. Adult groups who may need additional warm-up before personal disclosure may benefit from starting with check-in questions about their character, and then choosing to share about themselves as the bonus challenge.

Sample Check-In Questions

- *What is your favorite hobby or pastime?*
- *What is a talent you have?*
- *What is the weirdest thing you have ever eaten?*
- *If you could travel anywhere in the universe, where would you go?*
- *What is your favorite way to celebrate a special occasion?*
- *What is something you are proud of?*
- *What is something you have overcome?*
- *What is a skill you want to learn?*
- *What is your favorite childhood toy?*
- *What is a memory you cherish?*
- *What advice would you give yourself 5 years ago?*
- *What is something you look for in a friend?*
- *What is something you are afraid of?*
- *What is some advice you would give your character?*

Check-in questions should increase in depth, or opportunities for vulnerability, over time. Facilitators should use more personal questions, and questions targeted to support insight, as group cohesion and participant willingness increases. When increasing the challenge of check-in questions, facilitators should be mindful of the emotional impact on participants. If a more vulnerable check-in question challenged the players' stamina, a lighter, easier to answer question may be appropriate for the following session.

Additionally, check-in questions are intended to warm players up for the therapeutic delivery of experiential gameplay, not to be a majority of the session, so facilitators must be intentional about the time spent in the check-in process. There may be check-in questions that elicit enthusiastic personal sharing and elicit breakthroughs in peer reciprocity. When this happens, the facilitator must weigh the benefits of prolonged discussion against potential violations of group gameplay expectations and tactfully transition participants into gameplay when appropriate.

Check-In Activities

While check-in questions provide a safe participation structure for participants who benefit from clear performance expectations, some groups may benefit from occasionally having more active experiences during this time, especially for younger participants who may struggle to be present for the entire session. However, check-in activities should still be designed as a warm-up or to enrich the gameplay experience. Examples of check-in activities may involve art/craft activities (i.e., "draw your character"), embodiment activities (i.e., "walk around the room as your character"), or role-play activities (i.e., "interview another character").

Story Recap

After the check-in process, the participants transition into the gameplay portion of the session by collectively recalling the story progress from the previous session. This process can be aligned with the goals and needs of the particular group, as the purpose of the recap is to warm up and prepare the group more than to accurately recall every story beat from the session prior. Some facilitators may choose a particular participant to share what they remember from the previous session, while other groups will benefit from engaging in a shared participation structure.

Recap Technique: The Story Conductor

The GM pulls from their game kit a magic wand (or a dry-erase marker endowed with make-believe). "This is my magic story recap wand," they say. "When this wand points at you, your job is to recall exactly what happened last time we played. When the wand stops pointing at you, you will stop speaking—maybe even mid-word! When the wand points at the next person, they will continue our recap, maybe even finishing the previous person's word! Let's see how well this wand works!" The GM points it toward themself, begins with "Last time, in our adventure . . ." and then points the wand at a player who continues the recap.

Gameplay

While the check-in, recap, and check-out parts of the session are essential to the Game to Grow Method, the gameplay portion of the session is the core of the intervention, with each story encounter aligned with group goals and real-world areas of growth. Some gameplay sessions will be exhilarating, some will be challenging, and some players may struggle to participate. GMs are encouraged to trust the process (see Restraint, Chapter 12). The section on DOTS, later in this chapter, provides a clearly defined narrative structure to guide design of gameplay sessions and a framework for incorporating therapeutic goals into the story.

Check-Out

Where the check-in process is designed to "warm up" the participants, the check-out process is intended to "cool them down," support their insight and integration of gameplay content, and to leave the session regulated and eager to return. The check-out process involves asking each participant three questions:

- *What is a spotlight for someone else, something another player did that enhanced the game experience?*
- *What is something that was challenging or something you learned?*
- *What is something you predict or look forward to for the next time we play together?*

These three questions each provide an important opportunity for participants to engage in a reflection process, provide some feedback to the group, and to leave in anticipation of the next session. In order to reflect and validate the player experience, the facilitator may choose to repeat or re-state participant answers to these questions with an affective expression. The facilitator should also reply to the three check-out questions themselves, offering their personal reflections as both a model and an opportunity to highlight additional moments in the session.

Spotlight

The first check-out question encourages participants to express gratitude for each other. This may be a simple compliment or a profound appreciation. For participants who are less comfortable providing unsolicited positive regard, the structured prompt of a spotlight encourages development of group rapport and reinforces pro-social interactions and risk-taking.

Challenge

The challenge question is sandwiched between two more positive questions, as it is the opportunity for participants to share something that was personally difficult for them. They are invited by the question itself to frame their challenge as a learning opportunity, though participants will generally benefit from the facilitator reframing their challenge, validating their experience, and providing additional support. Some players may choose to share their frustrations with other players or with the game itself, which can be a valuable opportunity to support peer reciprocity and build self-advocacy skills. This is also when participants will reveal what kinds of additional support they may need. A participant sharing "I found it challenging to share my ideas" may be revealing a key opportunity for support and skillbuilding. Facilitators are encouraged to ask follow-up questions to elicit elaboration and cultivate additional insight.

Prediction

Because continuation desire is so integral to TA-RPG, ending with something the participants are looking forward to is immensely valuable. This provides a cushion after the participants share their challenge to verbalize their investment in the story of the game. Additionally, players will reveal their interests and their hopes for the story. Attuned GMs will take note and even include their ideas in future sessions!

Group Processing

Some degree of group processing will occur in every TA-RPG group, though if the group is a counseling group (as opposed to a social flourishing group) the session will conclude with a formal group processing component. All TA-RPG groups will have small moments of mid-session processing when appropriate. This may occur during the game by "pausing" the narrative in response to emergent issues, either mid-encounter or between encounters, to facilitate intra-group communication. Midgame processing should almost always be very brief, as to not interrupt the flow of the group or disrupt the narrative immersion. It should also be facilitated as close to the emergent moment as possible, though it is prudent in some circumstances to allow a narrative event to resolve before intervening if such a delay allows for deeper engagement in the therapeutic process.

The processing component of counseling TA-RPG groups is where relevant story content and in-game experiences can be brought to a group discussion via traditional group psychotherapy methods. In the processing portion of the session, the facilitator will scaffold peer-to-peer communication in order to encourage group-led discussion, validate the emotions and the experiences of the participants while managing vulnerability and supporting authenticity, and explore insights that players have gained into their personal lives through their experiences around the table.

When processing, group members are encouraged to reflect upon their personal experiences within the group and their character's experience within the game. For example, a game session provides an opportunity to experience a scenario targeting the needs of one or more group members (e.g., reading social cues, frustration tolerance, problem solving), while the discussion component allows for group members to review successes and failures within the game and process developing insights as a function of their in-session experiences. By shifting focus between players and their characters, the facilitator can guide insight and bridge valuable connections between the two. Over time, the accumulation of such experiences facilitates increased confidence and psychological flexibility.

Transition Rituals

While there are four or five sections of the session itself, there are also transitions between each of the sections, as well as transitions in and out of the session itself. In each transition, time and focus can be lost if the facilitator is not guiding the transition smoothly. Certain populations of participants may struggle to stay focused and may become dysregulated without clearly structured transitions from one activity to another. The more ritualized (i.e., repeated the same way each time with clear intentionality) these transitions can be, the better. When the facilitator uses not only the same participation structures but also the same words, tone, and cadence, the participants know exactly what to expect and can move seamlessly between activities.

The DOTS System of Narrative Construction

A Sandbox on Rails

Some GMs build entire worlds for their players to explore, at times spending hours designing aspects of the world the characters may or may not ever explore. This "sandbox" approach allows players the opportunity for open-ended exploration, completely deciding how their characters will interact with the game world. This approach can lack story continuity, as there are no constraints to exploration. Other GMs design very rigid storylines, often pressuring players to make specific choices to move the story they have created forward. This approach, known as "railroading," can limit player autonomy and prioritize the GM's design choices. GMs have debated the relative value of the two approaches, creating an unnecessary false dichotomy. With an understanding of narrative construction, GMs can align the game with a story while still retaining and rewarding player autonomy. The DOTS system of narrative construction, "a sandbox on rails," is a simple structure that honors the foundational story of the game while supporting the open-ended nature of the collaborative experience. Such a structure has many access points for designing encounters with therapeutic impact.

The DOTS system of narrative construction breaks down the game experience into individual scenes, called "encounters," that each have four components:

- Desire
- Obstacle
- Tactic
- So Then

Desire

The characters in a plot-driven story generally have a clear object or outcome that they desire. Sometimes the characters want to acquire a specific item, such as an amulet to lift a curse. Sometimes they want to achieve or prevent a certain outcome, such as throwing a cursed item into a volcano or preventing the re-emergence of a powerful villain. Without a desire, a tabletop role-playing game story has no plot, and the players will "sandbox" without purpose, wandering and exploring to find something that interests them. The first step to ensure the game has a story is to ensure that there are clear desires in every encounter, as well as in the story as a whole.

Desire Versus *Motivation*

The object or outcome that the characters desire is the physical, observable outcome of the plot. The reason *why* the characters desire the outcome can be left to the individual players to determine. If the heroes are questing for a valuable hidden treasure, their *desire* is to acquire the treasure. Their *motivation*, however, may be entirely unique to each player and their character. One player may want to be renowned as a famous treasure hunter, another may want the wealth to purchase new weapons to make them more powerful, and another may want to donate their new riches to the monastery that trained them. It is worth discussing with players not only the outcome of their quest but also the reason their characters are engaged in the quest at all. Ensuring both the players and characters are motivated by the story will help encourage buy-in and reduce some potentially interfering in-game behaviors. For more details on this, see "Collaborative Worldbuilding" in Chapter 11.

Obstacle

If characters were able to easily achieve the object or outcome they desire, the story would not be very interesting! For a story to have narrative tension, there must be a chance that the characters will not meet their goal, taking the form of an obstacle. This obstacle is what stands between the characters and their desired outcome. Sometimes the obstacle is a literal physical obstacle (e.g., the tunnel path is blocked by a massive boulder), sometimes it is a villain or adversary to overcome (e.g., the enemy forces refuse to let the heroes leave the castle safely), and sometimes it is an interpersonal obstacle (e.g., the town curmudgeon is the only one with the necessary information for the heroes to proceed). For more details on this, see "Encounter Types" in Chapter 10.

Tactic

The Desire and Obstacle are the pre-set aspects of the story. The tactics are comprised of the protagonists' actions and achievements (e.g., how they choose to overcome obstacles). In tabletop role-playing games, the players decide what actions their characters take, each character having their own unique skills, abilities, and resources to implement. GMs can plan or prepare for what tactics they may expect players to choose, and can even align tactics with treatment goals (see "Using DOTS Intentionally" in Chapter 10), though the tactic is always up to the players. Preserving player autonomy is essential to maintaining player engagement and allows the simulated nature of the game to feel responsive to player choices.

So Then

Not every tactic the protagonists use to attempt to overcome an obstacle in order to reach their desire will be successful. This is what makes a story have narrative tension and what makes tabletop role-playing games so exhilarating. After each character's attempt to overcome the obstacle, there is some kind of result, be it success, failure, or anywhere in between. As the GM describes the outcome of the player's choice, the desire is either met, not met, or has become closer or farther away (see "The Spectrum of 'Yes'" in Chapter 11). If the attempt is unsuccessful, the GM will describe the results of their attempt, offering to the players an opportunity to choose a new tactic. If the players are successful in their attempt and achieve their desire, the plot progresses and the GM will verbalize the transition to the next encounter, complete with its own desire, obstacle, and invitation to devise tactics. Building a story is as easy as connecting the dots.

DOTS Big and Small

DOTS are not just useful at the level of the individual scene. The four components of DOTS in a plot-driven story—Desire, Obstacle, Tactic, and So Then—can be identified at multiple levels of the plot. The DOTS of the campaign, and the subsequent adventures, will have in themselves many individual outcomes the protagonists desire, and the tactics they take may additionally be broken into subsequent DOTS. DOTS exist at the campaign level, adventure level, session level, and encounter level. There are DOTS in every CASE.

Table 10.1 Outlines Examples of DOTS (Desire, Obstacle, Tactic, and So Then) at Different Narrative Levels Including Campaign, Adventure, Session, and Encounter

Campaign	D: Dismantle the secret criminal organization known as "The Ring."
	O: The Ring is a powerful organization with branches all across the kingdom and agents in positions of power.
	T: Gain access to the membership list and make it public.
	S: The organization's criminal endeavors are stopped as its members are revealed and criminally charged by the authorities.
Adventure	D: Infiltrate the Westwatch branch of The Ring.
	O: The Westwatch organization only allows entrance to notable treasure hunters.
	T: Retrieve the lost amulet of Harlbrand and use it to gain entrance to the Westwatch branch. S: The heroes learn the location of the main headquarters of The Ring.

(Continued)

Table 10.1 (Continued)

Session	D: Learn the location of the amulet. O: Nobody currently living knows its location. T: Explore the library for archival history of nearby magic items. S: The heroes learn that the amulet is in a temple that sunk at the bottom of Lake Yarm
Encounter	D: Access the forbidden books section of the library. O: The door to the forbidden books area is trapped and will sound an alarm if there are trespassers. T: Cause a distraction, silence the alarm, or find another way into the room. S: The heroes swim to the bottom of the lake and find the temple.

Equipotential and Equifinality

Two important narrative concepts built into the DOTS system are equipotential and equifinality. A TTRPG story with equipotential is one that has multiple avenues to success at any level of DOTS. An encounter with equipotential has more than one successful tactic that will allow the protagonists to overcome the obstacle and reach their desire. For example, an encounter that involves crossing a rickety bridge may be open to multiple potential tactics (e.g., fortify the bridge, find another way across). An adventure or campaign with equipotential will have multiple successful strategies for success. As an example, if a campaign involves securing a prized possession from a monarch, the players have a plethora of strategies: Steal the item, trade it for a favor, blackmail the ruler, etc. When GMs plan encounters with one "correct" answer, such as a riddle with one answer, they are limiting the equipotential of the encounter, which may slow down story progress, frustrating players and hindering group development. However, when encounters have equipotential and players are able to choose from a nearly endless multitude of strategies and tactics, their creativity and engagement can be more readily cultivated.

When encounters, adventures, or campaigns have equifinality, the end result will always be the same regardless of the tactics employed. When GMs plan encounters with equifinality, they are not limiting player choice or restricting autonomy. Players are still able to think creatively and collaboratively though the story will progress in a semi-linear fashion informed by player decisions. For example, an encounter in which the players must enter a castle has equipotential and equifinality. The GM can prepare in advance for multiple tactics, knowing that eventually the players will enter the castle regardless of whether they sneak in through a window, hide in a delivered parcel, disguise themselves to infiltrate with the sentry, etc. Considering equifinality when using the DOTS system reduces planning burden on GMs and supports the integration of therapeutic content, as outlined in the following.

Enhancing Encounters

Encounter Types

Depending on the type of obstacle in the encounter itself and the expected tactics the players may use, it may be an exploration encounter, a combat encounter, or a role-play encounter.

EXPLORATION

With the exploration category of encounters, the obstacle or objective is related to the environment. This could not only include literally exploring an area, but may also include working to uncover or solve a puzzle, or navigating a situational hazard (i.e., scaling a wall, traversing a river, or escaping from a locked room). Players often must rely on creative problem-solving skills, and may use their character's abilities related to athletics, strength, and knowledge of the area/environment to help them progress.

COMBAT

In a combat encounter, the obstacle is a non-player character (NPC) or monster that must be defeated through physical or magical combat.

Table 10.2 Examples of Desires, Obstacles, and Tactics across TTRPG Encounter Types

Encounter Type	Desire	Obstacle	Expected Tactic
Exploration	Enter the forbidden book section of the library through the trapped door.	Physical obstacle in the world	Sleuth around the librarian's office to locate the secret trap door
Combat	Escape the forbidden books section unscathed after the dreaded Book Wyrm attacks!	A monster or villain	Fight with weapons or spells.
Role-Play	Leave the library in peace after the commotion in the forbidden books room.	The librarian	Convince the librarian it was an honest mistake.

Many TTRPGs center around dangerous fantasy worlds where combat plays a significant role within the game and setting. Combat often involves an increased number of defining rules, and more dice roles determining outcomes than exploration or role-play encounters, though this can vary significantly depending on the TTRPG being played. Players may use their character's weapons, spells, abilities, items, or creative uses of the environment to move forward. Combat often gives a space for players to support one another, and to think tactically about their character's abilities.

ROLE-PLAY

Similar to combat encounters, with role-play encounters, the obstacle is typically an NPC or a monster. However, in a role-play encounter, the tactic used to move past this obstacle is different. Instead of the use of physical aggression or magic spells to subdue or defeat the NPC, the players will attempt to engage in discussion with the NPC, and convince or trick them in a way that gets the player characters closer to their goal. Players may use their character's skills in persuasion, deception, intimidation, or other communication-based skills. In a role-play, the GM may encourage players to enact out the scene, having them say out loud what their character would like to say while the GM role-plays and portrays the NPC in the same fashion. In this way, role-play encounters can become a dialogue exchange between players and GMs who are each acting as a character within the story. Often, in a role-play encounter, players are trying to resolve conflict, gather information, or persuade the character/monster to aid the party in their quest.

A dynamic tabletop role-playing game experience will feature all three encounter types, as each contributes to the richness of the collaborative storytelling experience. Some players will naturally prefer certain types of encounters more than others, and GMs are advised to plan sessions accordingly. However, GMs are also encouraged to include all three with regularity, as each supports player engagement and growth in unique ways.

Shifting and Mixing Encounter Types

Because the DOTS system retains player autonomy, even if an encounter is intended to be a specific encounter type, player choice may shift a role-play encounter to a combat encounter or vice versa. Responsive GMs will follow the players' lead and let their choices guide the development of the story. Players may want to provoke a combat or talk an enemy into a truce, and this initiative should be honored as much as possible. While most encounters will have a primary encounter type, they will frequently feature aspects of other encounter types as well. For example, a combat may feature a villain verbally challenging the players (i.e., prompting role-play) or an exploration encounter may involve monsters being summoned (i.e., prompting combat).

Quantum Quandaries   GMs can build the spectrum of yes into the design of their encounters. Instead of planning an exploration encounter with all of the precise details predetermined and successful tactics pre-established, GMs can design "quantum quandaries," an encounter type which leaves additional aspects of the scenario open to player inquiry. Many encounters are open-ended challenges which provide the players multiple opportunities for tactics. Using the example of the players exploring how their characters will cross a rickety and unsafe bridge: One of the players may want to investigate whether they can fortify the posts embedded on the edge of the bridge. A GM who has designed this encounter as a more linear puzzle may answer with a simple "yes" or "no" depending on their preparation. A GM leveraging the spectrum of yes in a quantum quandary will allow the scenario itself to change in response to player interest. The GM may reply with a "no, but" or a "yes, but," such as "No, the ground is too loose and dry here to get the posts re-anchored, but you do see beneath the bridge some stones you could potentially tie some rope to," or, "Yes, it looks like the posts can be fortified, though you may need the help of an ally (referencing another character's strength) to really secure them deeply in the dirt."

Tone

Each encounter in a tabletop role-playing game, like a scene in any other type of story, has an emotional tone. When planning sessions in advance, the GM can plan the overall tone of the encounters for the session, aiming for some to be "light" in tone and some "dark" in tone. Light encounters are intended to increase the mirth, revelry, and feeling of hope in the story—the belief that the protagonists are progressing closer to their desire or are fearlessly facing the challenge. Encounters that are dark in tone can be somber, sad, frustrating, or otherwise provide some doubt that the heroes will accomplish their objective. It may seem counterintuitive to cause despair in players, but providing appropriately scaffolded challenges allows for successes to be more rewarding and for players to gain insight and experience the value of accomplishment through adversity. For more, see "The Impact of Affect", Chapter 11.

Accordion Opportunities

When designing encounters for a session with time constraints, it can be immensely helpful to plan for specific moments that can be expanded and/or contracted to meet the time needs. Such moments are considered Accordion Opportunities. GMs can plan ahead for where the session will ideally end and use Accordion Opportunities to maintain engagement while soaking surplus time and/or truncating encounters without the players feeling shortchanged. Additionally, identifying Accordion Opportunities can be incredibly valuable when players show an increased level of engagement during an encounter. If they are leaning in and collectively enjoying the moment, the GM should expand the experience by adding complexity or intrigue. This may require another encounter to be compressed. Thus, planning encounters in advance, with attention to each encounter's potential accordion opportunities, will enhance a GM's flexibility in facilitating an engaging session.

Ending on a Cliffhanger

Because participants' desire to continue participating is such a valuable aspect of TA-RPG, it is helpful for GMs to close each session with players eager to return to the following session. One way to accomplish this is for GMs to end sessions as they describe the conclusion of one encounter and the transition to the next—the So Then leading to the next encounter's Desire and Obstacle. When players are provided the opening encounter description at the end of the session, they have something to think about and prepare for during the time between sessions, allowing the game to stay with them even though they are not actively playing.

Scaffolding

Because the Game to Grow Method is both Developmental and Scaffolded (see Chapter 5), the degree to which players are challenged must be both planned in advance and adjusted in response to emerging player needs. Players show up to each session bringing with them emotions, mood, and thoughts informed by the rest of their context and lived experience. GMs who know their players well can anticipate in advance the appropriate level of challenge, but attuned GMs will adjust the challenge in the moment to meet the immediate needs and goals of the participants. Similar to planning accordion opportunities in advance, each encounter may also be prepared with opportunities to be more or less challenging in order to meet participant needs.

Tale From the Real-World Table

The GM prepared a challenging combat encounter, well-adjusted to players' previously assessed frustration tolerance. The protagonists were to battle skeletons that automatically re-assemble themselves upon defeat until the heroes re-assemble a collapsed statue. This encounter encouraged players to build their capacities of Regulation and Collaboration, and was ideal for the players' goals. The GM planned to have more or less skeletons in the combat and more or less parts of the statue as accordion opportunities. However, on the day of the particular session, some highway construction caused horrible traffic, resulting in several of the players arriving late and dysregulated. The attuned GM scaffolded the encounter to meet players' needs, by reducing difficulty and adjusting the tone of the encounter to be lighter. The skeletons, which were previously grim and menacing, became slapstick—their bones clattering off the walls upon defeat and only requiring one successful hit to be destroyed instead of several. The players felt collectively triumphant in their victory, never knowing that the original encounter was more difficult or feeling that the encounter was made easier because they weren't able to manage the challenge.

Integrating Therapeutic Goals With Session Content

Using DOTS Intentionally

When designing DOTS in alignment with treatment outcomes, consider ways the DOTS structure can support a goal held by an individual and/or the group. There are many ways to leverage DOTS to support growth. A therapeutic GM can align encounters with Core Capacity goals, promote insight through narrative transference when encounter elements are analogous to lived experience, promote new ways of thinking and acting by prompting and celebrating specific tactics and participation methods, and can provide much-needed access to feelings of triumph and levity by adapting tone and challenge level to meet player needs. Additionally, Yalom's 11 therapeutic factors in group therapy that support the effectiveness of TA-RPG (as outlined in Chapter 9) can inform encounter design and be supported by the DOTS framework.

Core Capacity Alignment

The Core Capacities of Regulation, Collaboration, Planning, Perspective, and Pretend Play are infused throughout the TA-RPG experience and can all be accessed and enhanced by virtue of engagement in a well-played game. However, GMs can plan in advance to focus on a specific Core Capacity in each encounter to meet players' goals for growth. As an example, the bridge encounter (Chapter 15) may be ideal for developing the Planning capacity, as it requires players to think logically about how to fortify the bridge and sequence their actions. However, the same encounter can be leveraged for Regulation, as the players may never feel completely confident of the safety of their crossing. Further, it could be leveraged for Collaboration, as cooperation between players will increase the odds of a successful crossing. While the encounter may be able to support growth in many Core Capacities, the way the GM facilitates the encounter will be targeted to the specific players on the specific day.

Analogous Desire/Obstacle

When designing encounters for therapeutic impact, the therapeutic GM can include aspects in the Desire and Obstacle elements (the elements built into the encounter that do not require player input) that are analogous to participants' real-world experience. It is essential that GMs not simply replicate sensitive content (e.g., traumatic events), but are harnessing the simulated nature of the game to introduce something analogous—distanced enough from reality to provide insight without dysregulation. As an example, a player who is working on impulsivity may have their character encounter a trap in the game where a much-desired object is protected by a powerful trap. While they will likely not encounter a literal trap around a literal magic goblet in their actual life, the challenges of and the consequences for impulsivity both in the game and from fellow participants may be analogous to their journey navigating impulsivity in their everyday experience. The opportunity for the player to experience and reflect on the analogous situation in a safe and distanced context can be leveraged for new insight and the development of new skills to navigate real-world situations.

Similarly, "navigating the unexpected" is a common life experience, as is "feeling stuck." These experiences can be conveyed in TA-RPG through unexpected in-game surprises or encounters where the characters must escape a perilous situation. An encounter where the protagonists are trapped in a room slowly filling with lava (see the "Tale From the Real-World Table" in Chapter 12) can feel analogous to a player's lived experience of an unexpected social encounter with family or a pop quiz at school. The players may instantly connect the encounter to their lived experience, though the facilitator may also prompt the connection and guide conversation during post-game processing.

When players interact with NPCs in the game, the NPCs and their interaction styles may be analogous with other individuals in the players' social microcosm. The players may struggle with their parents, an employer, or another authority figure in their lives. In the game, their characters may encounter a powerful noble who speaks over them, barks commands without consideration, or engages in manipulative insincerity. Navigating the analogous NPC provides an opportunity for insight into their personal response to the character and prompts group conversation about shared struggles with authority.

Encouraging Specific Tactics

When designing encounters analogous to real-world experiences, GMs may similarly align encounters with specific tactics they would like to prompt. The presentation of the tactic can be a literal skill of benefit to the player, or a symbolic representation in the simulation of the game. The GM must recognize that tactics which may benefit the participant can be encouraged, rewarded, or coached, and then scaffold the encounter in response to support player growth.

The example of the player navigating an in-game trap analogous to their own struggle with impulsivity (featured earlier) is not only an opportunity for insight and self-awareness but also one for practicing skills. Once the player experiences the struggle inherent in the encounter and becomes dysregulated, the GM can leverage aesthetic distance to narratively describe the character—as opposed to the player—as struggling. The GM can encourage the player to choose tactics for their character to navigate the situation, such as supporting their development of self-control, delay of gratification, planning, or reliance on teammates. By allowing the player to choose tactics for their character, they externalize the struggle with impulsivity, allowing an opportunity to witness both the impact of the impulsivity and successful practice of a tactic or a coping skill.

The DOTS system also provides a structure to support development of interpersonal effectiveness skills and a broadened repertoire of social tactics. The aforementioned "overbearing noble" encounter may prompt an opportunity to practice specific self-advocacy skills and values clarification. In such encounters, the success criteria for moving past the obstacle should be scaffolded and aligned with individual players' needs and goals. Players who are emerging in their comfort with self-advocacy need not execute the tactic perfectly, but can be successful simply by attempting a new tactic. Providing them encouragement and a feeling of success in self-advocacy will support their capacity development in the performance dimension (see "Three Dimensions of Capacity Building," Chapter 8). For players developing in the fluency dimension of capacity building, additional scaffolding and coaching may support the integration and generalization of a tactic.

Building conflict resolution skills is possible through intentional encounter design by creating encounters in which the players can practice either resolving conflicts between themselves and an NPC (such as in the aforementioned example) or between NPCs. In such an encounter, the obstacle may be that two NPCs argue or otherwise engage in conflict that prevents the characters from progressing. The Desire component of the encounter becomes "Get the NPCs to stop arguing and help the protagonists." When the players are presented with the challenge of helping NPCs navigate and resolve conflicts, the conflict is twice externalized from the players themselves. The conflict is taking place in a simulation, and it is occurring between characters portrayed by the GM. This level of distance with an externalized conflict may help players conceptually understand the conflict and support their development of skills. They could suggest a social tactic to an NPC (e.g., validate the other person's feelings) that they may not perform themselves (i.e., coach the NPC), observing the success of the tactic portrayed in the story. The players' modeling of adaptive conflict resolution skills in the moment, as well as the reflection back to the players that they chose a successful tactic, will support the development of the player's understanding and internalization of the skill.

In addition to conflict resolution and other interpersonal effectiveness skills, strategies to support the Core Capacity of Perspective can also be encouraged through the Tactics component of intentional encounter design. The players' characters may be blocked by an NPC, such as a guard preventing entrance to a fortress or a phantom who has trapped the protagonists in a cavern. In such an encounter, the players must interpret, understand, and respond to the "inner world" of the NPC in order to proceed. Because the GM is likely physically portraying the NPC with affect, as well as describing narratively their demeanor and actions, and because the players have the ability to ask questions and use the mechanics of the game to gain insight and aid their interpretation, the GM can scaffold the encounter to intentionally target the emerging skill.

A therapeutic GM designing encounters for their specific players may anticipate a range of tactics and success criteria depending on the needs of the specific individuals in the group. Many players will default to the use of the social tactics of threatening, intimidating, or otherwise coercing NPCs when they encounter NPC-based obstacles in the game.

Sometimes players who exhibit this tendency have a limited repertoire of interpersonal tactics and could be supported by the GM to build a broader range of prosocial interpersonal effectiveness skills. Other times, the player chooses antagonistic tactics as an experiment in power fantasy or an emerging expression of willful self-determinism. In such a situation, the GM may choose to allow an antagonistic tactic to be successful so that the player playfully experiences the positive reward of attention, the confidence boost of success, and the humor of the social interaction.

Some encounters may encourage players to give advice to an NPC on the basis of their own lived experience. This type of encounter allows a player to be an expert in their own lived experience without needing to face it directly as themselves or their character. By proxy, they may give themselves some positive self-talk. A player who struggles with self-acceptance may encounter a ghost whose unfinished business (i.e., the thing needed for them to reach eternal rest and thus let the characters progress in the story) is related to their guilt or shame. Because the NPC is analogously mirroring an aspect of their lived experience, when the player tells the ghost, "You're okay. It's okay, you did your best," they are invited to validate their own experience and witness how the NPC is liberated by self-acceptance.

Similarly, an NPC requiring advice or support may exhibit some of the maladaptive interaction styles of the players. When the players coach the NPC in adapting or adjusting their interaction style and witness them being successful, the players have an opportunity to speak aloud and be "the experts" in something they may struggle to exhibit in their own lives. As an example, a shy player may be enlisted to help a shy NPC who must advocate for themselves to a superior. The NPC may mirror some of the player's self-doubt and lack of confidence. Instead of the player having to practice confident presentation and advocacy, they may be able to tell the NPC how to stand, how to speak, and even coach the NPC in how to present their case.

Promoting Styles of Interaction

Outside of designing an encounter to analogously reflect a player's lived experience or promoting a specific tactic, GMs can design encounters specifically to promote a specific type or style of interaction and engagement. These encounters do not specifically require an in-game tactic that is generalizable (e.g., self-advocating to a superior or using coping skills to resist temptation), but support player growth by encouraging a type of interaction or engagement from the individual players as they engage in a collaborative game.

A combat encounter, for example, can serve multiple functions and should be leveraged by a TA-RPG facilitator mindfully. They are not meant to be included to either encourage literal violence or simply to increase playful engagement. In many TTRPGs, combat encounters require players to take turns. Turn-taking requires patience, focus, and executive function. Using a combat encounter to support the growth of these skills allows the GM to encourage and reinforce them without resorting to direct instruction. Players are more successful and more engaged in TTRPGs when they are skilled turn-takers, so the GM can reinforce skill acquisition very seamlessly.

Combat encounters also require players to rely on each other in unique ways that can be leveraged for player growth. The act of liberating another player's character who has been restrained by an enemy is an expression of trust and camaraderie. When a player's character is knocked unconscious and revived by another player's character, the two players engage in a vicarious recognition that they value each other and are willing to show it. For many individuals, the recognition that their presence matters and is valued by other group members is a cherished experience.

An encounter in which the players must concoct, discuss, and refine a multi-step strategy together requires listening, advocacy, and other collaboration skills. When the players are presented with the need to steal a treasured item from a moving train without the train conductor ever knowing, they are incentivized to turn to their fellow players and come up with a plan. This type of player-to-player interaction supports acquisition of interpersonal effectiveness skills, and the Collaboration capacity, especially when the GM reinforces their collaboration by describing the in-game results with active affective engagement. Players can collectively witness, in their imagination and around the table, the fruits of their collaboration and use the resulting positive feelings to encourage future collaboration.

When designing encounters with high-stakes narrative storytelling in mind, the GM can leverage the tension to invite players to engage in valuable perspective-taking skills for their own character. Simply asking "How is your character feeling right now?" provides a touchpoint for building emotional literacy and valuable content for future conversation and discussion. These in-game moments can be leveraged for insight into characters' complex inner worlds, their conflicted internal states, and the values conflicts that may be present. When a player reflects their character's distress, sadness, anger, or another unpleasant emotion, the GM can ask if and how the player's character shows their feelings externally (i.e., their affective display), what type of support they may need, whether they ask for support, and if they do, how the request is made. Rooting this entire interaction in collective narrative storytelling and using the tool of aesthetic distance, the GM can allow the player to externalize the unpleasant emotion onto their character to gain insight and to experiment with new responses.

Outcomes

When designing encounters using the DOTS system of narrative construction, the consequences of player choice—the "So Then" component of the encounter—can also be planned intentionally for player growth. Players may need to feel a sense of triumph, challenge, motivation, levity, etc., and with that in mind the GM can build an encounter to achieve a specific outcome. Regardless of the story content and the tactics the players choose, the GM can leverage the encounter to support a specific outcome.

In a social encounter, the desire is a revelation or resolution with another character. If the intended outcome is for a player to feel socially confident, the tactic may be inconsequential. A GM can instill the sense of social confidence and positive relational play by allowing their tactic to be successful regardless of how analogous or otherwise related it is to an ideal real-life social tactic. For example, if a social encounter featured an NPC blocking a path forward, a player may use a wide range of social tactics. Unlike an encounter in which the GM plans specific tactics to encourage, in an encounter focused on the outcome in mind, the GM can role-play the NPC in whichever way that would provide the player the intended result. If the player chose to intimidate the NPC, the GM can playfully cower in fear. If the player chose to boast to the NPC or to appeal to the NPC's better nature, the GM can adapt and respond to allow the player to see how their confident social tactic influenced the outcome. Sometimes players need to feel powerful, recognized, and celebrated for their contribution.

Similarly, encounters can be built with a focus on frustrating or challenging outcomes. In an encounter designed to build frustration tolerance, the GM may intentionally plan for "so then" content to be a long, uphill battle. Sometimes even great ideas fail, and even the best intentions can face unfair setbacks. When a GM sets up encounters with this in mind, the players are able to experience the vicarious frustrations of their characters and have the experience of confronting the challenge with a team of supportive allies.

Incorporating Yalom's 11 Factors

As outlined in Chapter 9, Yalom's 11 factors (i.e., Instillation of Hope, Universality, Imparting of Information, Altruism, Corrective Recapitulation, Development of Social Skills, Imitative Behavior, Interpersonal Learning, Group Cohesiveness, Catharsis, Existential Factors) can be cultivated by TA-RPG facilitators to support participant growth. Considering the 11 factors when designing encounters using the DOTS system, therapeutic GMs can ensure their incorporation and guide participant progress toward goals.

Intentionally planning the encounters' Desire and Obstacle with Yalom's factors in mind, therapeutic GMs can leverage existential factors by infusing opportunities for values-based decisions into moments of collaborative problem solving and can support altruism by encouraging heroic deeds. Through the intentional design and incorporation of NPC dynamics, therapeutic GMs can facilitate factors of universality, instillation of hope, and corrective recapitulation.

When encouraging players to use specific tactics to overcome an obstacle or promoting specific styles of interaction, GMs can leverage several additional of Yalom's factors. Imparting of information, development of social skills, imitative behavior, and interpersonal learning can all be leveraged through intentional facilitation of participant interaction and engagement with NPCs. Facilitators can provide direct support, scaffold peer instruction, and guide peer modeling. GMs can also support the factor of catharsis through encouraging authentic expression of emotion during role-play and peer interactions.

When building encounters with specific outcomes in mind, therapeutic GMs can consider the factor of group cohesiveness. When a group successfully achieves a goal together, navigates a difficult intragroup conflict, or experiences a shared moment of joy, the group will strengthen. With that goal in mind, GMs can be flexible about which tactics are individually successful because the overall outcome most beneficial to the group will increase the strength of the cohort.

Post-session Reflection to Guide Future Planning

After the session is over and participants leave, the therapeutic GM should take notes using the treatment planning and case conceptualization guides in Chapter 8. Valuable content to record will be the story events that occurred in each encounter, as well as player and group treatment progress. Salient content that emerged in the session should be noted, as it may be valuable to address in the future. When planning the next session, facilitators are advised to begin by reviewing the previous session's notes to see which story elements to emphasize, as well as which players may need extra attention, guidance, and support. Notes of which players received spotlights during the check-out process, which players struggled, and what emerging relationships could be leveraged in subsequent gameplay sessions.

The GM should also note their own subjective experience to inform and improve future processes. Was preparation adequate to meet the needs of the participants? Did the GM over-prepare for specific outcomes that did not manifest? Did the players surprise the GM with tactics they did not expect? If so, how did the GM respond? Were the participation structures well-aligned with player goals and adapted to their needs?

This personal reflection allows the therapeutic GM to continually hone their abilities to better serve their clients.

Conclusion

This chapter outlines the breadth of intentionality that can be infused into the design of a TA-RPG session. The individual sections of the session, and the transitions between them, are each planned in advance in alignment with individual treatment goals and the needs of the group as a whole. The DOTS system of narrative construction supports TA-RPG facilitators to be engaging GMs who lead cohesive and meaningful stories that respond to player input, and the framework provides opportunities to intentionally incorporate therapeutic intention into the many levels of the story.

11

Facilitation Strategies in the Game to Grow Method of Therapeutically Applied Role-Playing Games

The Game to Grow Method of Therapeutically Applied Role-Playing Games (TA-RPGs) is a synthesis of theoretical foundation, intentional preparation, and in-the-moment techniques that facilitate participants' growth. This chapter covers facilitation strategies to respond to challenges and support the intentional session design outlined in Chapter 10. These techniques support player engagement, encourage insight, and leverage the concepts outlined throughout this book. Additionally, this chapter outlines collaborative worldbuilding techniques to give players increased opportunity for investment in the experience.

The Silverware Technique

Gameplay can slow down or stall in TA-RPG sessions for a multitude of reasons. Such events are inevitable. Common causes of stall outs include player anxiety or distraction, interpersonal conflict between players, and a lack of a clear desire or obstacle in the encounter. When this occurs, facilitators are encouraged to use the silverware technique, consisting of offering a fork, spoon feeding, or twisting the knife.

Offering a Fork

When engaging in collaborative storytelling, some players may be confronted with anxiety as they ponder the seemingly infinite number of responses to a prompt. One way to alleviate this anxiety is to "offer a fork;" for the game master (GM) to provide a clear set of choices from which the players can choose. For example, instead of asking a player open-ended questions such as "Where is your character from?" a GM can reduce potential anxiety by asking the alternate question: "Is your character from a big city or a small town?" A similar anxiety may be prompted when players decide tactics to overcome an in-game obstacle. GMs can offer forks to aid in decision-making and empower players to move the story forward. For example, as players struggle to decide how

DOI: 10.4324/9781003281962-11

to enter a walled-off swamp town inhabited by dangerous adversaries, instead of the GM asking "How do you want to enter?" they can offer a fork by saying something like "Do you all want to go past the guard at the gate, climb over the wall, or find another way in?"

Offering a fork can also be a useful tool to support players who are boundary testing. Providing a set of options can offer implicit messaging about boundaries and offer clear options for the player. Offering the choice between befriending and intimidating an NPC implicitly removes the choice of attacking them. This tool can be useful out of the game-play portion of the session as well when redirecting participant behavior, especially for younger participants. For example, if a participant is playing with a distracting toy (i.e., not a regulation tool), the facilitator can provide the choice between putting it in a pocket and placing it on a table across the room.

Spoon Feeding

When helping players make decisions or move the story forward, offering a fork is a great first step that maintains player autonomy in their character's choices. When greater scaffolding is needed to support regulation, reduce anxiety, maintain narrative flow, or compress narrative sequencing for time constraints, the facilitator can "spoon feed" the players. Spoon feeding is when players are offered a clear next step or path forward. Adept GMs can veil spoon feeding behind guided questions or in-game moments. For example, when the players are prompted to rescue the NPC Sheamus in the Critical Core module The Little Town of Tusk, instead of the GM saying "Sheamus is hurt. What do you do next?" they can ask "How will you find a cleric to help you heal Sheamus?" Likewise, GMs can give selective information to players that prompt narrative momentum: "You see the clearest and easiest path to be through the front gate. Do you want to go there now?"

Twisting the Knife

The third tool in the silverware technique involves prompting player action by using an in-game situation to raise the narrative stakes. Players get distracted or disengaged for a variety of reasons, and instead of addressing the distraction or disengagement, facilitators can encourage players to reinvest in the story. GMs can incorporate a reminder of the overall plot, such as an NPC emotionally lamenting to the protagonists about the villain's most recent evil deed. The players' witnessing of the catastrophe they are working to resolve or prevent may remind them of their characters' overall desire. Similarly, if players are struggling to decide how to enter a castle in which their dear NPC companion is being held, the GM can use their affect to indicate to the players that they must act. The players may stop arguing about how to enter the castle once they hear the GM describe how they hear the sounds of their friend crying out for help.

The Spectrum of "Yes"

GMs are widely encouraged to "yes, and" their players, borrowing the concept from improvisational theater. In improv theater, one performer makes an offer to another performer in an improvised scene (e.g., "Dad, wake up! "You're supposed to take me to school today! We're late!"), and the other performer accepts the offer and expands upon it (e.g., "Oh, no, son! I slept in! Help me find my shoes!"). Improvised scenes are created as performers continue to accept and expand upon each other's contributions. This tool is essential in collaborative storytelling as the stories twist, turn, and shift with player input (not to mention when groups are engaged in collaborative homebrew, see later). The translation of the "yes, and" concept into TA-RPG encourages GMs to *accept* player choices (i.e., to acknowledge the player's contribution, not to confirm its success) and then to *expand* upon them. In other words, there are many more responses when players attempt to overcome obstacles than a simple "yes" or "no."

There are roughly six options for GM responses, ranging from extreme success to extreme failure. Using alternatives to "yes" and "no" move the story forward, reward player choice, and add excitement to even unsuccessful attempts.

Table 11.1 Outlines Possible GM Responses to a Scenario

Scenario

The protagonists need to get into a cave deep in the Viney Woods, but the cave entrance is covered in vines that are completely frozen over. (This is encounter four in the example module in Chapter 15.) One player decides they will charge at the vines and bash through them with their shoulder.

Response	Explanation	Example
Yes, and . . .	The attempt is successful and has an additional benefit.	The frozen vines shatter! The path is clear for the entire party to enter.
Yes.	The attempt is successful.	A crack appears in the frozen vine barrier large enough for one person to squeeze through.
Yes, but . . .	The attempt is successful, but has a small setback.	A crack appears in the frozen vine barrier, but the noise may have alerted nearby enemies.

Scenario

The protagonists need to get into a cave deep in the Viney Woods, but the cave entrance is covered in vines that are completely frozen over. (This is encounter four in the example module in Chapter 15.) One player decides they will charge at the vines and bash through them with their shoulder.

Response	Explanation	Example
No, but . . .	The attempt fails but has a small benefit.	A small crack appears in the vine barrier that could be pulled or wedged apart with some help from another character.
No.	The attempt fails.	The vines are too thick and the bashing has no effect.
No, and . . .	The attempt fails and has an additional setback.	The character slams into the frozen barrier and is now tangled up in the vines!

Rarely are "yes" and "no" responses the most interesting. Often, the most engaging gameplay comes from providing players with setbacks or new challenges to overcome. All of the "and" and "but" responses are built very directly on the specific input of the player, helping them feel like their contribution has a unique impact on the story.

Pronouns and Aesthetic Distance

Participants in TA-RPG groups will fluctuate in their aesthetic distance (further discussed in Chapter 5) with their character. At times, players will experience close aesthetic distance (i.e., over-identification) or remote aesthetic distance (i.e., under-identification) with their character. Player/character identification at various points on the aesthetic distance spectrum will be therapeutically valuable, depending on player goals. The therapeutic GM can expand or collapse the player's aesthetic distance by selectively addressing the player and the character.

To extend the player/character distance, the GM should differentiate between the two by referring to the character by the character's name or through a phrase such as "your character," which will externalize the character from the player and allow the player to consider their character thoughtfully. This can support the regulation of a player who often becomes emotionally dysregulated (i.e., in close aesthetic distance) when their character struggles or fails. With more distance between themselves and the character, the player may be able to make a clearer decision about their character's next action than when they are confronted with their own failure to succeed.

Likewise, when players experience a remote aesthetic distance and the attuned therapeutic GM wants to collapse the player/character distance, they can use the second-person pronoun "you" to do so. A replacement as simple as "Your character hears the sound of footsteps" with "You hear the sound of footsteps" can be incredibly useful to achieve stronger emotional resonance or encourage more narrative immersion. Notably, when players are playing aspirational characters, the therapeutic GM's use of the second person to contract player/character distance can help players internalize character successes into their own self-concept.

> You push as hard as you can and despite the odds you heave the boulder out of the way just long enough to save the villagers from the rushing water. They look at you with admiration and one of them rushes forth to hug you. "You were amazing!" a villager says with tears in their eyes.

Blurring the Lines

As the TA-RPG playspace is liminal (see "Play-Based" in Chapter 5), a player's identification with their character will fluctuate over time (and at times during a single session). The therapeutic GM is advised to embrace and encourage liminality by blending the use of second person and the character's name to link the two concepts, for example, "Blagdorf, what do you do next?" This way when the GM refers to Blagdorf in the third person in the future, the player will consider the reference to both them and their character simultaneously.

The Impact of Affect

Because the Game to Grow Method of TA-RPGs is at its core relational, the GM must be thoughtful and intentional about how they hold and manipulate their physical presentation in the interpersonal space of the therapeutic role-playing game (RPG). The therapeutic GM's affect— their facial, vocal, or bodily behaviors that indicate emotional expression and prompt emotional resonance—has an incredible ability to increase engagement and provides a valuable co-regulative function (Kret et al., 2013). Effective therapeutic GMs will understand the impacts of and be able to manipulate the multiple dimensions of their affect to meet player need and align with group goals.

Tomkins (1962–1991) outlined nine inherent affects that are experienced and displayed by infants and continually expressed throughout the lifespan: interest-excitement, enjoyment-joy, surprise-startle, fear-terror, distress-anguish, anger-rage, shame-humiliation, dissmell, and disgust. The hyphenated affects are named using the mildest and most intense end of the spectrum for that particular affect. Each affect has a specific physiological expression and a communicative function directed at others. A caregiver's attuned responsiveness to the affect display of an infant has been hypothesized by Basch (1983) as the foundation of empathy. This innate affective resonance, the ability of two individuals to connect on a subconscious level because of their individual affective experience, is core to the therapeutic GM's construction of their own affective display. A facilitator's capacity to recognize and relate to participants' affective display and to intentionally shift their own affective display is a valuable tool in the therapeutic GM's toolkit.

Players will often co-regulate with the GM due to their role as the session's guide. This may be particularly likely if the GM is facilitating a group session for individuals with relatively lower degrees of power and authority (e.g., age and cultural status). These power differentials exist regardless of whether they are acknowledged by the GM. Because of the unique position of the GM in setting the narrative tone and conducting the collaborative storytelling experience, their affect has the power to adjust the tone and experience of the story more than any one player alone.

The participants can perceive, interpret, and respond to the affective display of the GM as they facilitate the session, either to narrate the opening of an encounter, describe results of character action, or answer questions. The facilitator's vocal qualities—their speed, volume, pitch, the use of intentional pauses—may indicate emotional arousal and increase or decrease the inherent stakes of the narrative moment. In this case, the GM is very much like a radio announcer or emcee, responsible for cultivating the emotional response in the listener. The same applies for the embodied affective expression: facial expression, eye contact, gesticulation with the hands, whether the GM leans forward or back, stands or sits, etc.

Effective therapeutic GMs plan ahead for the tone of each encounter, recognizing the ideal narrative impact of each in-game situation. Many GMs improvise descriptions, but if they are aiming for emotional resonance it may help to plan out any specific phrases, pauses, and tone of delivery ahead of time. If the players would benefit from increasing the narrative stakes, maximizing the emotional resonance of a story moment to catalyze narrative transference, the facilitator should plan ahead to shift affective display accordingly: Increase vocal volume and enlarge physical affective display for an exciting dramatic moment or reduce volume, slow down, and lean forward to increase the dramatic tension. If the players need a lighthearted moment to increase emotional and cognitive distance with the story and reduce tension, the facilitator may plan for a more subdued affective display of enjoyment-joy. The GM should use the same toolset to describe what happens when players take actions. They can be exciting, tense, silly, sad, gross, etc. Likewise, an attuned therapeutic GM will perceive, interpret, and respond to the affective display of the participants and shift their own affective display. If the players are emotionally aroused and becoming dysregulated, either by narrative transference or because of other situational factors, the GM's reduced affective display can help the participants co-regulate and reduce the emotional arousal. Moments of perceived chaos in the narrative or in the shared playspace can also become dysregulating to some players, and they will likely take cues from the affective display of the GM. If the GM responds to these moments with an affect display of interest-excitement or enjoyment-joy, the players can co-regulate with this cue and reduce their own emotional arousal, perhaps even experiencing these positive affects for themselves. Of course, a flat affect is also a powerful tool! Use a flat or minimal affect when players need to co-regulate and reduce tension.

Use Affect as a Carrot

The use of affective display is not only valuable as a tool for running effective games, but is also incredibly helpful at facilitating the group before, during, and after the gameplay portion of a session. Whereas a visibly nervous-looking facilitator may cause participants to feel dysregulated, a facilitator's warm and calm affect can contribute to participant feeling of safety. Similarly, an enthusiastic response from the facilitator who appears authentically interested in a participant's answers to a check-in question will support participants' feeling that their responses have value. The goal of utilizing facilitator affect in this way is not to provide extrinsic rewards but to allow for participants to experience the positive intrinsic experience of having their unique contributions celebrated.

Bend, Accordion, and Shift

Many GMs are encouraged to bend or break the specific rules of a tabletop role-playing game (TTRPG) system according to the "rule of cool," in which a priority is placed on that which is exciting or cinematic for the players over the rules as written. When facilitating TA-RPG groups, we encourage facilitators to employ a slightly modified version of this rule called "The Enthusiasm Doctrine."

The Enthusiasm Doctrine:

You can bend or break whatever rules you want because your true goal as a game master is to encourage vivacious whole-brained engagement in authentic relational play!

Always remember the rules are there to *support* the group's engagement in play. If there are rules that are instead inhibiting the facilitator or their player's ability to engage enthusiastically in authentic relational play, we encourage facilitators to adapt, suspend, or replace those rules! GMs should feel empowered not only to bend or break rules but also to expand or contract attention and time dedicated to specific encounters and to even shift the game's entire direction to meet player interest, engagement, needs, and individual goals.

Bend or Break Rules

Facilitators should first decide how important it is to follow the specific rules as written. GMs should be selective when applying rules with a high likelihood for player confusion or a low likelihood for player success. While most TTRPGs have a formal set of rules and guidelines to determine player success, the GM may need to bend or break rules intentionally (and at times secretly) to choose the degree of a player success aligned with player growth. Additionally, because the rules of the specific TTRPG system may instruct the GM to leverage dice rolls or implement rules in opposition to character's interests (e.g., rolling dice for monster attacks or limiting character movement). Therapeutic GMs are empowered to selectively lie on dice rolls or to "fudge" the rules when appropriate, though players should still have an air of mystery around GM machinations to maintain sanctity of the simulation. When appropriate, such fudging of numbers can include topics such as the number of hit points left on a monster, the inner workings of a trap, or even the number of zombies present in the next room.

When deciding whether or not to fudge a roll or ability check, the facilitator should weigh the therapeutic goal costs and benefits. For example, if a client has a great idea for sneaking across rooftops to drop down and surprise a group of enemies, and their roll is borderline (could be a success or a failure) the value of each outcome should be examined. If the check succeeds, it will likely provide a boost to the client's sense of agency and self-esteem. It may also increase the character's competence in the eyes of the party. In contrast, if this is a client used to succeeding and is working on building frustration tolerance, a failure may be of more therapeutic value.

Accordion

GMs can and should spend extra time and place extra emphasis on encounters or situations that align with the group's ultimate needs and goals. If a player struggling to engage socially is having a full back-and-forth in-character conversation with an NPC who was originally intended to serve a short, transactional role, the GM can linger on the conversation and even have the NPC become important to the story in response to player engagement. Conversely, an attuned GM will sense when to compress (i.e., cut short) an encounter or activity that is not supporting players' progress. Instead of cajoling players to engage in an open-ended quantum quandary during a session in which players struggle to fully participate, the GM can provide a simple success criterion to move the story along and maintain engagement.

Shift Game Direction

Sometimes GMs must abandon their plans and shift the entire direction and plot of a story to meet their players. This may be in response to something aversive (i.e., altering any plague-focused stories at the onset of COVID-19 pandemic to avoid the uncomfortable topic) or something attractive (i.e., the players all expressed an interest in pirates after the release of a popular movie, so the GM incorporates seafaring and swashbuckling to encourage players to connect over a shared interest).

Making the Most of Non-player Characters

In RPGs, the non-player characters (NPCs) played by the GM provide a rich reservoir of engagement potential. They can be quest givers, bitter enemies, valuable allies, and comic relief. The variety of NPCs is only limited by the GM's imagination. GMs who use verbal and physical affect to make NPCs distinct from themselves will provide additional opportunities for engagement, narrative immersion, and personal growth.

What Is the NPC's Purpose?

When adding NPCs to a campaign, the GM should consider the purpose of the character and their contribution to the story's plot and impact on its narrative tone. Will they serve as an obstacle the heroes must overcome in the narrative, will they help the heroes in their quest, or is their purpose to influence the story's narrative tension? Perhaps both! When designing role-play encounters in which NPCs are used as obstacles preventing characters from progressing until the players use a successful tactic, NPCs should have some sort of motivation for blocking characters progress. Are they self-interested? Acting out of fear and self-preservation? Are they having a bad day and want to make life difficult for the heroes? Are they a lost soul bent on revenge? Obstacle NPCs without character motivations can cause the story to feel arbitrary, that the NPC is a puzzle to be solved instead of a narrative interaction to be enjoyed.

NPCs used to increase or decrease narrative tension should still have their own motivations to make them well-rounded characters, but because they are not serving as an obstacle the players must overcome to reach their desire, they need not be as clearly defined. A simple interaction with an NPC can enrich the narrative by reminding the players of the story's stakes and allow the players to experience the richness of the game world. An NPC with this function may raise the stakes of the story, such as the forest sprite in the Viney Woods (see the example module in Chapter 15). That NPC's function is to strike an emotional chord with the players and prompt them to action. Adding additional idiosyncrasies to NPCs can also enrich the world of the story, such as a particular style of dress or a mannerism the NPC uses as they communicate. NPCs for levity may be silly, buffoonish, or slapstick, usually intended as one-time interactions to boost player mood and lighten narrative tone, but sometimes players will become attached to these characters and request additional visits or even "adopt" them!

Tagalong NPCs

Sometimes, a GM will have NPCs tag along with the adventuring party as the story progresses. These tagalong NPCs may be included by player request, to support participant goals, or because the story being told requires this character to be present, but should not be included if the GM's sole desire is to feel included in the player experience. Some tagalong NPCs may even have their own character sheets with skills and abilities that can be used to overcome obstacles or assist in combat, but should never take the narrative spotlight away from the characters played by players. To accomplish this, the NPC can be designed with abilities that directly support those of the other players or with significantly less abilities than the heroes. GMs may also encourage players to discuss collaboratively what tactic a tagalong NPC should take in an encounter and then "convince" them to use it. Using tagalong NPCs can provide additional opportunities for the characters to build relationships and have additional opportunities for social interaction.

Using NPCs Intentionally

Regardless of the NPC's purpose, they are an important tool for therapeutic GMs. They can help set tone and encourage player engagement in the story, but when leveraged intentionally can provide many additional benefits that can prompt players to insight, growth, and change. Though not an exhaustive list of ways to utilize NPCs, the following list provides several examples of functions NPCs can serve.

Embrace the Whimsy

Role-playing NPCs, especially if the GM uses a clear physical embodiment and voice for them, can encourage players to lean into the play aspect of TA-RPG. Allowing them the opportunity for narrative transportation into make-believe will empower them to push boundaries, try new behaviors, and experiment with aspects of their identity.

Playful Irreverence

Because of the liminal quality of RPGs, GMs can speak through both themselves and NPCs. As such they can say things out loud that the GM wouldn't say, providing an opportunity for playful irreverence and some direct challenges to player behaviors. For example, when players are being rude or hostile to an NPC, a GM with enough rapport with the players may be able to push back playfully: "Oh, you think this is how you're going to get me to help you? Making demands without a care to me and my needs!? Do you think this is a good way to get what you want!?" The language used by this NPC is likely different from the tone the therapeutic GM would otherwise take with the player, so will probably get the attention of the players and prompt an in-character response. The ability to have this playful confrontation in character with some aesthetic distance can catalyze new insights.

Narrative Transference and Social Rehearsal

When players connect in-game scenarios to their real-world circumstances, they have an opportunity to use the analogous experience of the game to practice social interactions in a low-stakes environment. Players who in their out-of-game life may struggle with assertiveness and interpersonal effectiveness can practice new ways of social interaction through their character. For example, a player who is navigating a relationship with an employer or a parent may be able to project the situation onto an NPC interaction, practicing new ways to be empowered and assertive.

Guidance and Feedback

NPCs can create opportunities for facilitators to provide information to participants through avenues other than themselves. The facilitator can play characters like a grumpy guard, excited child, or patronizing librarian, all of whom allow the facilitator to provide guidance or feedback through proxies to support participant receptiveness. For example, if the players are all speaking over each other, the facilitator could embody the child character through a high-pitched voice, while covering their ears, and saying "You're all being too loud!" Alternatively, as the librarian, the facilitator could take a haughty and proper tone and demand that the characters "Leave my library immediately, and don't come back until you've found some manners!" Both of these NPCs function to support participants in receiving feedback about their behavior through the story. Further, because the facilitator wasn't the one directly giving the feedback (the NPC was), the facilitator was positioned to problem-solve *with* the players. Facilitators should be mindful of participants' responses to their NPC usage, as some participants may interpret the NPC's actions as indistinct from the facilitator's. This may be particularly likely with participants who struggle with perspective taking, or in situations in which the facilitator has not yet developed adequate trust with the group.

Social Dynamics

NPCs can shift group dynamics in a player group by altering the group's interpersonal connections. A participant who enters into the group with self-protective rejection behaviors may engage in antisocial or antagonistic behaviors because they expect the group to exclude them. Attuned therapeutic GMs responding to this situation can incorporate into the story an NPC who absolutely admires and respects their character. The player pushing to be rejected will not meet that outcome and their character will continue to be met with unconditional positive regard. Because the NPC is played by the GM, when the GM speaks for the NPC and directs their positive regard their way, the player can reciprocally receive the message that they are safe and welcome.

Similarly, a player group that is navigating the complexities of peer aggression may benefit from an NPC who can be the recipient of the group's ire, channeling the peer antagonism away from the group and aligning the group in solidarity against the NPC. This NPC could be a villain of the story, a nefarious opponent who thwarts the protagonist's quest and prompting their cohesion, or a particularly annoying tagalong NPC the group of heroes is stuck with. This type of character can be the same as the previously mentioned adoring character. An egregiously sycophantic tagalong NPC can simultaneously boost player confidence through effusive compliments and be the recipient of redirected playful antagonism.

A Tale From the Real-World Table

A group of teen players, who were struggling to collaborate, often belittling and demeaning each other's ideas, were joined by a three-foot tall gnome by the name of Mordnap Nimbletoes. The attuned GM had intuited that these players' social dynamic would benefit if they could triangulate their frustrations in real time against a silly NPC who could absorb all of their ire. Mordnap spoke in a high-pitched voice and was effusive with praise and admiration for the heroes. He was in constant awe of their triumphs, no matter how trivial, and whenever he could, he'd offer to play his pan flute (mimed poorly by the GM!). The players who used to argue with each other, each anticipating the rejection of their peers, became used to having Mornap around. They could all acknowledge Mordnap's sometimes frustrating social interaction patterns and practice setting boundaries with him. Mordnap filled an important role in the group such that the other players could collectively position themselves against Mordnap instead of each other. Though Mordnap was a seemingly constant source of annoyance to the players, they did not hate him. When Mordnap was kidnapped, the players immediately came to his rescue!

Collaborative Worldbuilding

Some therapeutic GMs choose to run their games using established materials and pre-written stories like those in Critical Core. There is an abundance of materials that have been made available for GMs to leverage in their groups. However, using a pre-written adventure without adapting it to the interests of the players may have some unfortunate additional consequences resulting from the lack of player buy-in. For example, many GMs report challenges with rampant destruction from players (sometimes called "murder tourism") who are not engaged with the story or world. This may stem from a perceived lack of agency or relevance to the participant. Using collaborative worldbuilding techniques will incorporate player interest and voice into the adventure, even if simply to modify the name or description of an NPC or location in a pre-written adventure. Limited choice methods are best for a quick low-stakes incorporation of player input, while open-ended methods are more challenging for players but rich in opportunities for engagement.

Limited-Choice Methods

When the players are first meeting an NPC or coming across a new location, the GM can have the players help name the NPC or location by inviting players to collaborate. NPCs or locations can be named one letter at a time such that each player adds a letter to the name resulting in a word no one could have built alone. The players work together to give the character a name, instilling a sense of collective ownership over that character.

When naming locations in the world, the GM can also prompt player input with a request for a part of speech, that is, requesting an adjective from one player and an animal from another. The characters can then experience the pleasure of eating at the "The Angry Heron," created by the input of the players.

Open-Ended Methods

When players are comfortable with invitations to collaborate, the GM can invite them to collaboratively worldbuild with more open-ended requests. The players may be asked to provide specific details of NPCs, locations, etc., such as "This NPC is wearing a distinct article of clothing. What is it?" or "The town you're entering is particularly known for a unique food item. What is it?" When the players then meet the NPC with the eyepatch or walk around a town where everyone is eating fried fish eyes on a stick, they see their input made manifest. Even better if GMs can leverage this collaborative opportunity to enhance a character, that is, "Blagdorf, you have been to this town before, what do you remember about it?" These can be interpreted as a "gossip," which means it can be interpreted as partially true without having to take the player's suggestion verbatim. A player who suggests that "everyone who enters the town gets rich" may have their character enter a town and be given an all-they-can-eat coupon to Rich's Fish Eye Emporium.

Benefits of Collaborative Worldbuilding Techniques

Incorporating collaborative worldbuilding techniques not only helps players have a sense of ownership over the story and the world but also encourages collaboration, creativity, and flexible thinking. Some therapy-interfering behaviors may also be reduced when players have an opportunity to have their voice heard in positive ways. Players who are exhibiting a strong desire for control, are boundary-testing, or otherwise lack engagement, may benefit from incorporating their voice into the story directly through collaborative worldbuilding.

Collaborative Campaign Creation

GMs can increase the benefits of collaborative worldbuilding by incorporating player voice and desire into the creation of the adventure itself. The process consists of the following steps:

1. Create a map.
2. Add "gossip" about map locations.

3. Create adventure hooks, called "rumors."
4. Vote on one rumor to be the basis of the story.
5. Embellish the rumor with additional gossip.

Creating a Map

Using a piece of paper, a dry-erase board, or a shared virtual whiteboard, the group will collaborate to build a map of unexplored territory: the location the adventure will take place. To create this map, each player will take turns drawing one geographic feature on the map without explaining or naming their contribution. After the group determines that the map is sufficiently full of features, the players can take turns naming items or using the collaborative naming methods outlined previously to name geographic features.

Adding Gossip About Map Locations

After the map is created, players take turns creating "gossip" about specific map locations by making up things their characters have "heard" about the locations, statements that may or may not be entirely true using an "I heard . . ." sentence frame. This gossip allows players to add mystery and intrigue to the map, that is, "I heard that the town of Eastwatch has a vampire problem," or to add some silliness "I heard all the teachers at the Magikram University literally have eyes in the back of their head." The "I heard . . ." sentence frame supports the players' understanding that the statements have questionable validity.

Creating Adventure Hooks, Called "Rumors"

Once the map is created and embellished with gossip, the players create adventure hooks, known as rumors, by creating three components: A bad thing that is happening or about to happen, a location on the map for the bad thing, and a reason why the characters care about resolving the issue. Depending on the group, players can write their rumors on paper and hand them to the GM or submit them electronically. Rumors may be related to the gossip on the map, but needn't be. Examples include:

*   The town of Trawnvail is attacked every full moon by werewolves. The mayor has offered access to the town's vault of magic items as a reward.
*   The kingdoms of Ralknam and Plamner are about to go to war. The rulers have each been lied to about the reasons for war by someone interested in putting the whole continent into chaos. We care because we want to save lives!

- Students are being kidnapped from Magikram. We care because we have to protect students!
- Long ago, pirate treasure was buried deep within Hopedust mountain. Whoever finds the treasure first will be entered into the Adventurer's Hall of Fame. We want to be rich and famous!

The reason the characters care about preventing the "bad thing" from happening may be motivated by a variety of factors (e.g., heroism, external reward). Allowing players to create their own adventure hooks empowers them to advocate for the type of story they want to play, be it a heroic battle against monsters for a reward, preventing war, or rescuing children. The pirate treasure hook from the aforementioned example isn't a "bad thing"—it's an "exciting thing" instead. Starting with the component of a "bad thing" can help provide some structure to support participants who struggle with creativity. When players are ready for more open-ended requests, facilitators can expand the rumor instructions.

Voting on One Rumor to Be the Basis of the Story

Once players have created rumors, players vote on which rumor they would like to be the foundation of their adventure. Depending on the group, players can discuss openly which they like and why, or vote anonymously. Allowing players to vote for their own in addition to others may be particularly helpful in reducing frustrations in younger players. There are many ways to vote, and GMs will decide which methods will be most appropriate for the group (i.e., online survey, index cards, show of hands).

Embellishing the Rumor With Additional Gossip

Once a rumor has been chosen (or an amalgamation of two or more rumors has been created), players will each create another "I heard . . ." gossip statement to embellish the rumor. This additional inclusion of player voice will allow each player to have a contribution to the main plot of the story even if their rumor was not selected by the group. This gossip must be related to the chosen rumor, but can incorporate aspects of their own interests that had not been chosen. Players should be advised to have their additional rumor gossip contribute to the rumor as opposed to derailing it.

Common Roadblocks to Treatment

Commonly identified challenges to TA-RPG treatment include participant behaviors such as disengagement, making negative comments about other group members, and acting in ways that are counter to group goals.

These behaviors disrupt the development of social competence and of rewarding and meaningful interpersonal relationships, which are the primary goals for many participants. Though these "roadblocks" may be frustrating to both GMs and players, they should be considered part of the treatment plan. These are not problems to be circumnavigated but are the treatment goals to be addressed.

Antisocial Behavior and Inappropriate Language

As with any therapy group, especially one targeting social skills, it is common to have participants display socially aggressive behavior. In addition to the goal for a client to reduce this behavior, the continued engagement of this type of behavior in session can erode the sense of a safe and trusting place where it is okay to make mistakes. In order to support these players, engage in functional analysis (Chapter 8) and support the player's insight by allowing the character to be the one engaging in the antisocial behaviors (see pronouns in Chapter 11). Additionally, use NPCs (see "Making the Most of Non-Player Characters" in Chapter 11) to provide opportunities for playful proxy feedback from the GM, social practice, corrective recapitulation, and to disrupt player–player aggression by introducing another character who can safely and playfully absorb peer aggression while the player adjusts to the social group.

Typically, the use of inappropriate language is part of normal limit testing in groups. The developmental level of the group as well as the group setting will determine what language is and is not appropriate for the group. Functional analysis will inform the GM with the potential intent of the inappropriate language, and the GM should do their best not to inadvertently reward the use of inappropriate language. Depending on the function of the behavior, if the GM responds either as themself or an NPC with insult, outrage, or aggression, the behavior may be reinforced. When these limits are tested, redirecting in a flat or reduced affect with "please make another choice" or "please pick another word" can set the limit firmly but gently.

Asocial Behavior

The balance between honoring player autonomy and maintaining narrative continuity can be difficult to manage when a participant plays their character as a "lone wolf" acting in solitude or openly refusing to engage in the adventure with the other players. Using functional analysis (Chapter 8), an attuned GM may infer that the player may be wanting control of the narrative, developing their capacity for collaboration and flexibility, and/or unready to trust other players to keep them safe. Refusing the player's choice to determine their character's destiny (i.e., refusing to allow them to go their own way) can cause conflict and disrupt the developing rapport.

If a player describes their character heading off on their own, they can, though the player can be reminded that the consequence is that they will be "off-stage" or "off-camera" when they do. This means that they will not get detailed descriptions or the same kind of engagement that the rest of the group receives. Additionally, because their character is not in the same location as the rest of the group, they will not be able to talk to the other characters. This means the client whose character has split off is unable to offer advice, give directions, or help with whatever encounter the party is facing until they return to the party. A player wanting narrative control will discover that they actually get less of what they want by splitting off on their own, and players developing their capacity for collaboration will be provided an opportunity to observe the benefits of working with allies or the consequences of thinking they can accomplish everything better alone.

Self-Protective Rejection of Others

Some players will develop an aggressive or negative demeanor in an attempt to push others away before they can be rejected themselves. They believe that rejection from others is unavoidable and engage in antisocial behavior to expedite the inevitable. This can be especially true among individuals who have experienced rejection or bullying. Prove them wrong! It is essential that therapeutic GMs identify this intention and do what they can to avoid allowing this behavior to be reinforced. Players exhibiting self-protective rejection behaviors need to feel accepted, safe, and included. Facilitators should respond to players with unconditional positive regard, redirecting, reframing, or ignoring antisocial behaviors whenever possible.

Backseat Game Mastering

Like a passenger in a car dictating or criticizing the way the driver of the car is driving, that is, "backseat driving," some players who are experienced with TTRPGs may engage in "backseat game mastering" by critiquing the GM or otherwise demanding the game to be facilitated in the way they expect. This is not a phenomenon unique to TA-RPG, and can be handled in much the same way as it would be in any other therapy group. With functional analysis (Chapter 8), the GM should work to identify which of the player's needs are not being met and if the observed behavior aligns with the player's treatment goals. For example, a client with a goal of taking turns and listening to others may have trouble listening while the therapeutic GM is speaking. Or, if the client feels more comfortable when they are in control of situations, the perceived power differential between clinician and client and between GM and player may be a struggle for them. Resolving these issues could take the form of establishing collaborative table guidelines and behavior expectations, or by helping the client take a clearly defined role as expert, that is, the official person to look up/recall rules when requested, the helper of less experienced players, etc. Additionally, the client may require increased knowledge or skills around successful communication or ways to help them interrupt less (i.e., taking notes for the party, writing down what they want to contribute, raising their hand when they want a turn to speak).

A Tale From the Real-World Table

Steve, an adolescent participant, created a character who behaved as a loner that didn't play well with others. He overtly expressed that he didn't want to work with the other characters, refused to share their knowledge to help them, and even tried to steal from them. While the player was allowed to have their character leave the group and follow their own path, the narrative focus remained with the other group members. Additionally, Steve quickly learned that when his character split away from the others, he forfeited any influence he could have over the group's actions.

While processing with the group after the gameplay portion of the session, Steve expressed difficulty working with others and regular experiences of rejection from peers. He described a history of experiences that taught him he didn't need other people. Further, Steve would anticipate rejection each time his character took actions that could potentially harm the party. Although other group members experienced and expressed frustration in response to this client's character's behavior, they continued to express acceptance of the client and his character within the group.

Once Steve began to trust that he would not be rejected, but was part of a team, he slowly began engaging in prosocial behaviors (i.e., collaboratively planning and acting, sharing, and complimenting) and began providing their thoughts and feelings regarding courses of action for the entire party. In response, Steve was praised for his behavior by other group members. Over time, he became more open to collaboration within the group, and his character began engaging in more prosocial behavior. Further, following his return from a break, Steve chose to create a new character that was intentionally designed to better support and coordinate with the group.

References

Basch, M. F. (1983). Empathic understanding: A review of the concept and some theoretical considerations. *Journal of the American Psychoanalytic Association, 31,* 101–126.

Kret, M. E., Roelofs, K., Stekelenburg, J. J., & de Gelder, B. (2013). Emotional signals from faces, bodies and scenes influence observers' face expressions, fixations and pupil-size. *Frontiers in Human Neuroscience, 7.* https://doi.org/10.3389/fnhum.2013.00810

Tomkins, S. (1962–1991). *Affect imagery consciousness* (Vols. I–III). Springer.

12

SPARK
Characteristics of a Great Therapeutic Game Master

Great therapeutic game masters (GMs) have that "special something." But what does it take to be a great therapeutic GM? Is it an encyclopedic knowledge of the game system's rules? Does it take years and years of personal experience as a player and GM before beginning professional practice? Following more than a decade of experience in providing therapeutically applied role-playing game (TA-RPG) and training the next generation of new therapeutic GMs, several themes have emerged. While dedicated study and gaming experience certainly help new GMs build their knowledge and skills, the in-session disposition of the therapeutic GM will have a greater impact on their success than years of dedicated study. Great therapeutic GMs possess a unique energy and in-the-moment responsiveness that allows them to be fully present, creative, and ready for anything.

Great therapeutic GMs do not just have a spark, they have SPARK:

- Spontaneity
- Playfulness
- Attunement
- Restraint
- Knowledge

Spontaneity

Great therapeutic GMs are fully present. They respond in the moment without being stuck in their heads or anxious about what will happen next. Spontaneity, an essential theme in psychodrama and many creative arts techniques (Malchiodi, 2003), is defined as "A state in which psychological energy propels the individual to act appropriately to an unpredictable situation without a second thought, inhibition, guilt, or self-doubt" (Moreno, as cited in Davelaar et al., 2008, p. 118). Jacob Moreno, founder of Psychodrama, also defined spontaneity as "the

DOI: 10.4324/9781003281962-12

adequate response to a new situation, or the novel [and adequate] response to an old situation" (Moreno, as cited in Sternberg & Garcia, 2000, p. 124). GMs, even recreational GMs, must be ready for players to think of new solutions to in-game obstacles for which they could never have prepared, or to take the story into new directions based on players' novel interests and curiosities. Therapeutic GMs must additionally be prepared not only to respond in the moment to unexpected player choices but also to respond to the emergence of salient opportunities for insight and growth.

All GMs must simultaneously hold the game structure, the overall story, and the players' subjective experience in their attention. Beyond this complex set of stimuli, therapeutic GMs must track additional factors while they facilitate TA-RPGs, including the management of participant goals and progress, as well as planned interventions to encourage continued growth in participants. This can be quite a lot to manage! New therapeutic GMs may struggle to attend to the multiple dimensions of the TA-RPG experience without becoming anxious that they may fail to execute all aspects of TA-RPG with aptitude. In fact, anxiety is described in sociodrama literature as "blocked spontaneity" (Sternberg & Garcia, 2000, p. 128). Anxious therapeutic GMs with blocked spontaneity may be more likely to rigidly adhere to rules or planned encounters, resulting in missed opportunities for player engagement and growth.

Building spontaneity takes practice. Therapeutic GMs are advised to regularly try new activities and experience being out of their comfort zone. Such practice may also increase compassion with clients who may be apprehensive to try TA-RPGs. It may be necessary for therapeutic GMs to gather with friends or colleagues to engage in spontaneity play, which may resemble children's playground games or improv theater exercises. A therapeutic GM's capacity to display spontaneity will also provide a valuable model for participants who may struggle with self-efficacy and self-esteem, both of which are positively correlated with spontaneity (Davelaar et al., 2008). Additionally, therapeutic GMs may benefit from "warming up" before a TA-RPG session. This process may include a physical activity to increase blood flow and help the facilitator feel more present, such as jumping jacks or dancing along to a favorite song. Another spontaneity warm-up, used for years by Adam D. Davis and Adam R. Johns, is the creation of a one-word-at-a-time improvised story. One facilitator would start with "Once," and the other would say "upon," and they would continue alternating back and forth until a story would emerge. The goal of such an activity is not to make a "good" story, but to respond with the first impulse and observe the story that emerges.

A Tale From the Real-World Table

The therapeutic GM originally planned a particular session's encounters to target the Core Capacity of Planning by having the protagonists explore a riverbank to investigate the mystery of an abandoned mine. The plan was to have them track clues, discuss the ties between the clues, and draw a linear conclusion based on logical sequencing. When the participants arrived for the session, one of the players lets the group know that they had recently experienced a seizure and would like their character to also have a seizure in the game. The therapeutic GM recognized the salience of this moment, adjusted their tone and demeanor, and shifted the encounter in the session to include a spontaneous seizure experienced by the character, the player's disclosure of a complicated medical situation, and the other group members' empathetic and supportive response both in and out of character. This shift was only possible because of the therapeutic GM's spontaneity—the receptivity and willingness to shift in the moment to meet the needs of the participants.

Playfulness

Great therapeutic GMs are curious explorers who never forget their role as a model and guide for many anxious or weary participants into the untraveled territories of play. The Game to Grow Method of TA-RPG is play-based (see Chapter 5), so it may seem redundant to state that great therapeutic GMs have the quality and disposition of playfulness, though this extra emphasis is important because of the many roles a therapeutic GM must fill during a TA-RPG session. The balance between facilitating a fun and engaging game experience and facilitating a session focused on participant growth and personal development can be difficult to manage. It can be tempting for therapeutic GMs to become so focused on achieving outcomes, or on reducing the occurrence of specific behaviors, that the game experience can become rote. Without play, it may make TA-RPG seem like a "gamification" of therapy as opposed to an authentically play-based intervention.

The Game to Grow Method is not a discrete skill training model, but a social flourishing model. A GM could prompt and reinforce target behaviors using in-game rewards and token economies, but essential to this intervention is a focus on authentic relational play. The group facilitator's embodiment of play, their genuine curiosity and enthusiastic engagement, is contagious and must be kept at the forefront of their mind. This modeling will help participants continue to develop their Pretend Play capacity, making the entire experience more engaging.

Similar to spontaneity, a playful disposition must be honed and practiced. The activities suggested to train spontaneity will also encourage a playful disposition. Therapeutic GMs are also advised to participate in recreational tabletop role-playing games (TTRPGs) as a way to maintain a foundational reference point for the fun inherent in the game format. When therapeutic GMs exclusively run TA-RPG groups, they may lose track of what it means to play and enjoy a TTRPG for its own sake.

A Tale From the Real-World Table

The therapeutic GM had been working with a group of adolescent participants for several months. They each struggled in school or community settings to form relationships, and the goal each of their parents had was for them to make friends and reduce antagonistic behaviors. The GM included a tagalong non-player character (NPC) to join them in their adventure: an annoying gnome bard named Mordnap Nimbletoes that could absorb the brunt of their peer aggression so they would not turn against each other. Many groups warm up to Mordnap and take him in like a little brother. This group sensed that Mordnap was a "tool" of the GM to help them make friends, not a "real" character in the fantasy game they wanted to play. One of the players declared, "When Mordnap walks away, I'm going to shoot him in the back with my crossbow!" Normally, the GM would redirect this type of action. The players knew this. The GM was tempted to pause the game and have a discussion about the importance of relationship building or reflect with the group on how their antagonistic behaviors were interrupting their ability to build trusting, supportive, relationships. Instead, the GM leaned into the play. The GM replied, "The crossbow bolt slams into Mordnap's spine. He crumples to the ground, dead as a doornail." The group looked wide-eyed at the GM, shocked that he actually let it happen. After a pause, the master described: "Slowly, a mist floats up from Mordnap's lifeless body. It swirls for a moment then forms the shape of . . . Mordnap." The players looked confused. The GM then assumed the wide-eyed countenance of Mordnap, patting himself on the chest and down his arms, then continued in Mordnap's high-pitched cartoon mouse voice: "Oh no! Somebody shot me! Who could have possibly done such a terrible thing!? We'll have to find out who did it! Wait . . . if I'm a ghost, this means I don't have to eat or sleep and we can now be together FOREVER!" The GM gave his players a mischievous look. Instead of being yet another adult telling them they were wrong or wanting to change them, the GM was someone willing to play with them. That particular group never did learn to love Mordnap, ghost or not, but they did develop a sense of safety and rapport with the GM that allowed for future conversations and reflections that would have otherwise been impossible.

Attunement

Great therapeutic GMs humanize their players, make personal connections with them, and allow them to share the lead. They "read the room," modifying their challenges and adjusting their affect in response to players' signals. When they are not able to intuit signals from players, they ask for clarification. Because the Game to Grow Method is both Relational (Chapter 5) and Scaffolded (Chapter 5), GMs who lack attunement will miss opportunities to develop player–facilitator reciprocity and player–player reciprocity, as well as struggle to identify when and how to introduce scaffolding to support player growth.

Attunement is the ability for therapeutic GMs to not only undertake in-the-moment perspective taking, but an active practice of flexibly connecting with the energy of players and the group as a whole. Attuned therapeutic GMs pay attention to player affect, the expression of emotion through how they hold their bodies and use their voices. They note expressions of tension (e.g., clenched jaws and furrowed eyebrows), as well as interest-excitement (e.g., leaning forward, raised eyebrows, elevated articulation of the arms), and determine how the affect response of the player supports their overall engagement and growth trajectory.

Using co-regulation, the GM adjusts their own affect in response to player affect. Attuned GMs can even engage in mirroring to boost feelings of belonging, a process referred to as "the chameleon effect" (Maddux et al., 2008). By using similar body language, phrasing, or expressions, as the participants, the GM can inspire participants' sense that they are seen as part of the same group. Similarly, the GM is encouraged to repeat back to the participant what they say during check-in and check-out portions of the session in order to both clarify understanding and show the participant that they are actively listening.

Several techniques in the attuned therapeutic GM's repertoire can assist in-the-moment assessment of player mood.

The Thumb-o-Meter

The GM asks each player to hold up their thumb somewhere in the range between straight up and straight down. This "meter" reflects the player's mood, their day so far, their energy level, etc.

Silent Check-In

The GM asks each participant to face the GM and place their hand up against their chest (ideally so that only the GM can see), either with a thumb up, meaning "I'm great," an "ok" symbol, meaning "I'm fine," or a flat wavering hand meaning "I am not okay."

HALT

The GM explains that HALT stands for hungry, angry, lonely, tired, and that each of those experiences can impact the way people engage in activities, even ones they enjoy. Players hold up one to four fingers to outline how many are impacting their day.

Each of the aforementioned techniques should provide opportunities for participants to convey what may be a complicated internal state without the use of spoken or written language. As players may have difficulty putting their emotions or context into words or feel challenged explaining themselves, they may be able to commit to a simple embodied response to a prompt that will provide the GM enough information to adjust to meet their needs.

Attunement occurs not only with individuals but also with groups. In his book *To Sell Is Human*, Dan Pink explores the concept of group attunement, and coins a process he calls "social cartography," which he defines as "the capacity to size up a situation and, in one's mind, draw a map of how people are related" (2014, p. 74). The ability for therapeutic GMs to conduct social cartography, similar to Jacob Moreno's (1953) "sociometry," provides an ability to understand how group members relate to each other. Recognizing the relationships within a group and their nature (e.g., which group members have positive rapport, which have negative rapport, which group members are leaders, and which are followers) can be tremendously valuable as GMs push groups to think, feel, and act in new ways.

A Tale From the Real-World Table

The GM began with the Thumb-o-meter. Three of the four players, comfortable in the group environment, showed a thumb straight up. Meanwhile, one new player, Chris, held their thumb sideways. The GM also noticed that Chris was shifting in their chair, looking around the room and at the clock. The GM interpreted that Chris was probably less comfortable than their sideways thumb would indicate, but that they may have been uncomfortable showing a straight-down thumb. The GM continued to pay attention to this player's signals, looking for the right moment to clearly invite them to shine. In the story, the protagonists were traveling through a magic swamp. The GM had prepared for the swamp to have either an exploration obstacle or a combat obstacle, depending on the energy and needs of the group. Another player, Kira, a natural leader in the group who was very comfortable taking initiative, announced that they would forge ahead into the swamp. Reading the room, the GM decided to start with an exploration obstacle: The carnivorous vines in the swamp would try to restrain the heroes, starting with the lead player who would find this exhilarating. The GM saw Chris continually watching and taking cues from the confident player, and decided to have Kira's character lifted in the air. The GM described the vine quickly grab the hero's ankle and pull them high into the air. The GM then said, "The vines are all over the trees so it looks too dangerous to climb up. You all may need to get them down from a distance." Kira, well-versed in the rules, knew that Chris' character was proficient with a bow and arrow. They turned to Chris and said "Chris! Shoot me down! Shoot me down!" Kira then helped Chris roll the appropriate dice to shoot the arrow and free their character from the vine. When their character fell into the mud, the GM described how it splattered over Chris' character and the two were now drenched in mud. They looked at each other and laughed. The GM noticed that the other two players, who had not yet acted, were looking at the other two players intently. The GM turned to them. "You two notice that Kira and Chris' characters are now well camouflaged since they're covered in mud . . . Anything you want to do about that?" The other two players instantly declared that they would roll around in the mud to also be camouflaged and to share in the moment. At the end of the session, Chris received spotlights from other players about their initiative to save Kira's character, how useful the camouflage was in the ensuing combat, and how hilarious it was when they were covered in mud. This moment was made possible because the GM paid attention to the signals of the players and sensed the relationships between them. The GM trusted that Kira would support and welcome Chris if given an in-game opportunity, and sensed that Kira's invitation to participate would be more evocative than a prompt from a facilitator.

Restraint

While spontaneity, playfulness, and attunement require therapeutic GMs to be active and engaged, great therapeutic GMs also trust the process, knowing not only when to lean forward and take the lead but also when to allow players to take the lead and even allow them to struggle just outside their comfort zone. Not every session occurs perfectly. Some may even go poorly! Therapeutic GMs must have the personal restraint to be gentle with themselves in the moment and as part of a reflective practice.

It is easy for therapeutic GMs to want to help players who are struggling, or to take the reins when the group is off-track. A group may be distracted, descending into conflict, or struggling to overcome an in-game obstacle. Sometimes the instinct to be a helper must be restrained, and players must be afforded the experience to struggle, navigate, and learn on their own. While the GM wants players to succeed, they must scaffold appropriately to ensure participants have a sense of achievement for their victories. Sometimes, too much help can cause more harm than no help at all. The act of restraint is essential to resist the urge to help and support players when experiencing a challenge would be most aligned with their treatment goals.

It is common for GMs to put time, energy, and attention into planning their sessions, designing the world of the game, and plotting out the story. This personal investment supports the TA-RPG experience for all players, but therapeutic GMs must also hold a position of non-attachment to their creation, as they must abandon their masterpiece when the needs and goals of participants must be prioritized over the value of their personal investment. By allowing stories to be player-led, facilitators support the relational nature of the TA-RPG experience and support the participants in building the capacity of Collaboration, even if the facilitator's creation is a work of creative storytelling genius!

Some sessions occur perfectly: Each participant enjoys the session, progresses toward a treatment goal, and leaves eager to return. However, not every session is ideal. Sometimes, careful preparations manifest clumsily, joyous play seems foreign, and group members may openly critique or criticize the story or the facilitator. When this happens (and it will), great therapeutic GMs must have the personal restraint not to become overly self-critical. The position of non-attachment is essential to GMs resisting the urge to take control of the narrative and "railroad" the players, as well as allowing GMs to be reflective without succumbing to self-defeating criticism.

To become a restrained therapeutic GM, one that is responsive instead of reactive, build a reflective practice. Being restrained as a therapeutic GM will be easier if the practice of mindful self-observation is a practiced habit both in and out of session. One must resist the immediate desire to react, reflect on opportunities to harness potential for growth, and make a decision to respond in the best interests of the participants.

A Tale From the Real-World Table

The GM set her players up in an encounter which was going to require them to work together. The players, all adolescents, were working on building social confidence and had all had expressed struggles with building friendships at school. Each was very comfortable playing online games with friends, but had a low tolerance and comfort level with conflict. When they would argue or disagree with online friends, their tactic was to turn off the game and do something else instead of navigating the disagreement or resolving the conflict. In the game session, the protagonists were placed in a situation in which they were all trapped in a room that was slowly filling up with lava. There was a pedestal in the center of the room that would potentially allow them to escape the lava and even escape the room, but they would need to work together to climb the pedestal and safely avoid the lava. The players each had their own unique plan to avoid the lava, sometimes suggesting tactics that would guarantee another player's character would not survive the incident. Naturally, conflict arose. The conversation became heated and the GM felt the urge to point out (using the Spoon feeding technique, Chapter 11), the relatively simple potential solution to this situation, that if they would only collaborate, they could easily avoid the lava! Instead, the GM let the players struggle. The players had not experienced a conflict that they actually wanted to navigate, but now, because they cared about their characters and they cared about their collective story, they wanted to push through their discomfort with conflict and asked the GM for help. The GM did not provide the solution to the encounter, as much as she wanted to, but helped the players talk to each other, express their ideas, and ultimately to collaborate. If the GM had stepped in when she felt the impulse to "rescue" her players, they would not have had the opportunity for a valuable corrective experience and one that became a foundation for future growth. The therapeutic GM had noticed a personal desire to save her participants from discomfort and to guarantee their success in the encounter. However, with the power of self-observation, she was also able to trust the process and let the players take the lead.

Knowledge

A great therapeutic GM is knowledgeable within several domains. They must possess a rich knowledge of their therapeutic interventions, the game system being used in the TA-RPG session, and the participants' goals, contexts, and interests. While every GM must be adequately prepared with knowledge about the story and the world of the game, therapeutic GMs must also prepare before sessions to ensure in-game scenarios are aligned to participant areas of growth. A comprehensive reflective practice is essential for therapeutic GMs to self-assess knowledge deficits and identify opportunities to continue improving.

Great therapeutic GMs must be adequately trained in both their intervention and in the populations they serve. When therapeutic GMs are not adequately trained, they can cause harm just as in any other therapeutic intervention. It is essential for therapeutic GMs to act within the ethical bounds of their training, and make sure participants are receiving the best possible care.

It is also crucial for GMs to possess adequate knowledge of the game system they are using in the TA-RPG session. While it is not essential to have memorized every variation of every rule, a foundational knowledge of the rules is important to maintain continuity of the game experience (e.g., not disrupting play to refer to rulebooks). Additionally, a GM who is unknowledgeable of the chosen game system will be seen by some participants as a betrayal of expectations and will slow group cohesion and rapport-building. Some participants, on the other hand, will be completely content or even excited to be the "expert" for therapeutic GMs who are not fluent in the game system's rules. For these players, this opportunity to be seen as knowledgeable and help the group will boost their confidence and support their growth. The GM can provide this opportunity to players regardless of if they actually know the rules. Thus, it is best to have a thorough understanding of the rules and feign ignorance when it supports participant and group growth.

A comprehensive intake process will help therapeutic GMs understand the complexity of each player: their goals, their challenges, the histories and systems that inform their context. When therapeutic GMs have not adequately assessed and learned about their participants, they could potentially cause harm or at the very least miss valuable opportunities for growth and insight. TA-RPG facilitators with a rich understanding of their participants will be able to make informed decisions about how to set players up for growth and success. Refer to the section on Treatment Planning (Chapter 8) for more about gathering and using information about participants in TA-RPGs. It will also be helpful for therapeutic GMs to gather information about a player's interests, the media they consume, and the hobbies they enjoy. A GM's ability to knowingly slip in a mention of a cherished cultural reference or to shift the game's content to include a player's interests will help players feel seen and promote increased engagement.

While a comprehensive knowledge of the therapeutic intervention, the players, and the rules will improve the effectiveness of TA-RPG implementation, each therapeutic GM must determine what level of session preparation is "adequate" for them and their players. When therapeutic GMs have not prepared for a session, they must rely more on their spontaneity and in-the-moment tools to conduct the session. Some GMs will have more success than others, as they are more comfortable with improvisation, but participants who sense that a facilitator is anxiously unprepared may respond with dysregulation, power struggles, or a decline in trust.

When great therapeutic GMs are confronted with a knowledge deficit, they address it by seeking additional resources, training, and consultation. If a participant brings up an issue in session that the therapeutic GM is not adequately trained to handle, they will seek consultation or refer the participant to other services until such a time that they are adequately trained to handle the situation. When a therapeutic GM observes a participant mention a favored activity or piece of media, they will seek to learn more about it to use it to strengthen their relationship. Great therapeutic GMs are continually reflecting on their skills, trying new approaches, and identifying ways they can improve.

A Tale From the Real-World Table

The therapeutic GM, who was fully trained in their therapeutic intervention and fluent with the rules of the game they were playing, was welcoming a new player into a running-enrollment TA-RPG group. The new player's parent shared that the new participant struggled with extreme social anxiety. They regularly missed days of school and refused to leave home. The GM also asked in their intake process about the interests of the player. The parent shared that the player spent a majority of their free time playing Minecraft, a video game in which players are able to collect resources from the environment and use them to craft and build weapons, equipment, and buildings. The GM knew that several of the other players had also mentioned Minecraft in passing, or as part of previous check-in questions, so the therapeutic GM assumed it could be leveraged to build group cohesion around a shared interest. The GM was determined to learn more about Minecraft and incorporate the themes into the TA-RPG game. They sought information about it via the Internet, asked colleagues about the game, and even borrowed a copy of the game to play on their own. When the participants arrived for their first session together, the GM began with the check-in question (see Chapter 10): "If you could build anything from scratch, what would it be and why?"

This question was chosen so that players would hopefully bring up their shared love of Minecraft, casually and without the GM's overt facilitation. They did! The anxious new player was now leaning forward, looking around the room at their new peers. Once the game started, the GM introduced the new player's character and gave them a powerful magic item: a magic wrench that could separate the components in mundane items and reconstruct them in new ways (a concept in clear reference to Minecraft). All of the returning players were excited about this new player, their magical ability to craft, and to have someone else to connect with about a shared love of Minecraft. This intervention was only possible because the GM collected rich information about client interests in the intake process, paid attention to the expressions of the other participants, and sought new knowledge to benefit the group as a whole.

References

Davelaar, P. M., Araujo, F. S., & Kipper, D. A. (2008). The Revised Spontaneity Assessment Inventory (SAI-R): Relationship to goal orientation, motivation, perceived self-efficacy, and self-esteem. *The Arts in Psychotherapy, 35*(2), 117–128. https://doi.org/10.1016/j.aip.2008.01.003

Maddux, W. W., Mullen, E., & Galinsky, A. D. (2008). Chameleons bake bigger pies and take bigger pieces: Strategic behavioral mimicry facilitates negotiation outcomes. *Journal of Experimental Social Psychology, 44*(2), 461–468. https://doi.org/10.1016/j.jesp.2007.02.003

Malchiodi, C. A. (2003). Expressive arts therapy and multimodal approaches. In C. A. Malchiodi (Ed.), *Handbook of art therapy* (pp. 106–119). The Guilford Press.

Moreno, J. L. (1953). *Who shall survive?: A new approach to the problem of human interrelations.* Beacon House.

Pink, D. H. (2014). *To sell is human.* Canongate.

Sternberg, P., & Garcia, A. (2000). *Sociodrama: Who's in your shoes?* Praeger.

13

Starting a Therapeutically Applied Role-Playing Game Group

Starting a therapeutically applied role-playing game (TA-RPG) group is an exciting experience, and well-prepared facilitators will accomplish much of the work to set the group up for success before the first participant sits down at the table (or logs into the session). When planning a TA-RPG group, it is vital to have a clear understanding of the intended goals of the group, the target population, and any organizational supports and constraints. Additionally, as group cohesion is positively related to treatment outcome (Bernard et al., 2008; Burlingame et al., 2011), facilitators must have a clear understanding of the factors that create a group with a high potential for cohesion. The screening process for TA-RPG group participants should address exclusion- and cohesion-related factors, and serve to set participants up with reasonable expectations for their participation in the group. Facilitators should be intentional about the structure of their groups, including size, parent or guardian participation, outcome monitoring, between-group activities, and the development of character sheets. When starting a group, facilitators need to be intentional in their introduction of safety tools, ensuring the methods chosen by the facilitator will be effectively utilized by participants.

Screening

When creating a new group, it is important to screen all potential members to determine their appropriateness to the intervention (i.e., assess for exclusion criteria and clinical contraindications), as well as their fit within the goals for this particular group (Frances et al., 1980). Although many individuals can be appropriate for TA-RPG groups, not all individuals will be appropriate for a particular TA-RPG group due to age, support needs, goals, or presenting symptomatology. Identifying the general age range, level of support, and broad group goals before recruitment can be helpful in recruiting and selecting appropriate group members.

The screening process for group members can typically be completed in 20 minutes, or may be conducted as part of a standard

DOI: 10.4324/9781003281962-13

biopsychosocial intake for mental health services. The two goals of the screening interview are to gather information about the participant and to set expectations for the intervention. During the screening interview, it is important to collect information about the participant's (and parent or guardian's if applicable) goals for treatment, potential risk or "therapy interfering" concerns, as well as the participant's experience with tabletop role-playing games (TTRPGs) and therapy. Useful information is shared not only in the language used in the responses but also in the ways the respondent replies and the information left unsaid or unaddressed.

Questions to ask

1. Participant and parent* goals
2. Potential risk
3. "Therapy interfering" issues
4. Experience with TTRPG and therapy
5. "No List" topics/triggers

Data to Gather

1. How does the participant speak about themselves/hobbies/goals?
2. How does the parent speak about the participant/goals/hobbies?
3. Does the participant have a regulation toolkit?
4. What does the participant care about?

Specific screening questions should be tailored to the type of group and setting—for example, for an in-person group, facilitators will need to confirm information related to physical supplies, transportation, and supervision expectations (i.e., if the parent will be expected to stay in the area). For virtual groups, facilitators should gather information about access to the necessary technology for group participation, such as a camera, microphone, and stable Internet connection. Also, facilitators should identify where the participant will meet for each group, and ensure appropriate confidentiality with consideration for potential risk concerns.

The screening intake is also a space to provide information about TA-RPGs broadly and the specific group to the participant. During this time, the facilitator can ensure they have a general understanding of the course of the group, including information about expected group size and enrolment norms (open, closed, or rolling admission). Participants should be informed about the amount of TTRPG knowledge they are expected to have before joining the group (usually none), and ask questions they have about TTRPGs or the group.

Exclusion Criteria

Currently, there is no evidence to suggest that utilizing TTRPGs in group interventions poses an increased risk with traditional group therapy methods. Two recent reviews of the literature on applied role-playing games (RPGs) did not identify areas of risk, but noted the research in this area is still emerging (Henrich & Worthington, 2021; Arenas et al., 2022). As with any therapeutic intervention, care should be taken when considering possible clinical contraindications. Additionally, the competence of the provider to work with a given population and the organizational supports available should be considered when determining eligibility for group participation. The following topics are a non-exhaustive list of possible exclusion criteria.

Reality Testing

Reality testing is an evaluative process wherein individuals distinguish their internal, subjective experiences (e.g., thoughts and feelings) from external, objective experiences. Clients who struggle with reality testing (e.g., individuals experiencing active psychosis) may be inappropriate for a TA-RPG group if they struggle to discriminate between self and others and between fantasy and real life. This should be examined on a case-by-case basis, as the nature of specific, active delusions or hallucinations may not necessitate group exclusion. The likelihood for effective participation in a TA-RPG group increases when there is evidence that clients are able to appropriately participate in and contribute to other psychotherapy groups. Further, clients who are able to safely consume media with fictional or fantasy themes, without exacerbation of symptoms, can likely employ similar strategies and successfully participate in a TA-RPG group.

Suicidality

Formal suicide risk assessment should be considered when clients, either directly or through their character, make comments related to suicide and self-harm, or express deep or persistent feelings of hopelessness (SAMHSA, 2020). Suicide risk assessment should generally be done one-on-one, outside of the group. Clinicians should follow organizational and state guidelines pertaining to safety planning and reporting if immediate risk to safety is determined. Suicidal ideation, independent of suicidal plan or suicidal intent, should generally not be treated as exclusionary criteria for participation in TA-RPGs. Further, suicidal ideation may be considered an indication that individual therapy may be an important adjunctive intervention to ensure proper care and treatment (Stone et al., 2017).

Violence

Individuals presenting active concerns regarding physical violence/ aggression within a group are not a good fit without extra consideration on the part of the clinician. For example, clinicians may employ behavioral contracts or utilize a co-facilitator that is responsible for de-escalating potentially volatile situations. In some circumstances, accommodations can be made that contextually reduce concerns related to violence/aggression when the client's triggers are removed from the group environment (e.g., altering variables such as light, sound, temperature, seating, group size). Facilitators should follow organizational guidelines and prioritize the safety of group members. Individuals with active physical violence concerns may be a good fit for virtual/ telehealth groups.

Disability

Disabilities should not be considered exclusionary criteria for most groups. TTRPGs are adaptable and benefit from their ability to accommodate physical and neurological diversity. More information concerning accommodation and inclusivity of clients can be found in Chapter 7.

Considerations for Group Cohesion

Diversity among group members is valued in TA-RPGs, providing clients opportunities to experience a wider range of perspectives than could be found within homogenous groups. An increased capacity to adopt others' perspectives is particularly relevant to clients with treatment goals related to deeper social engagement or broader social competency (Ragins & Ehrhardt, 2021; Weiler et al., 2013). Further, exposure to new experiences and opinions may challenge rigid thinking patterns with which a client presents.

Age

When creating groups for children and adolescents, it is advised to cluster participants within the same general developmental window. Though younger players may benefit from the modeling of an older group member, problems can arise when the developmental gap is too broad. For example, a significant age differential during adolescence may result in clients' feeling alienated from their peers. In contrast, a wide range of ages has been found to be clinically valuable among adults in TA-RPG groups, particularly when clients share a common background or other demographic variable (e.g., military veterans; Kilmer & Kilmer, 2018).

Diagnosis

As with many psychotherapy groups, diversity of both diagnoses and goals is encouraged within TA-RPG groups (Yalom & Leszcz, 2020). Superordinate goals and shared experiences within the context of the game can help to establish team-building and a sense of universality among a heterogeneous group. Additionally, across diagnoses, many clients have similar treatment goals regarding increased insight, frustration tolerance, communication, and conflict resolution skills, all of which can be addressed through TA-RPGs.

Informed Consent

Consent is profoundly important within any relationship. It helps to establish respect, trust, and expectations for future interactions, which serve as crucial components of any therapeutic relationship. Indeed, accurate client expectations have been consistently linked to better treatment outcomes, and this may be especially important in the context of unfamiliar and novel interventions (Greenberg et al., 2006). In the context of gaming, clear discussions around consent help to assure players that their experience in session will more closely reflect their expectations. For example, individuals who have experienced a traumatic event in their past and who currently experience distress when reminded of the event may prefer to limit in-game reminders of their trauma or otherwise triggering content.

Consent must also be a transparent process such that clients who enter into a therapeutic relationship are fully "informed" of the parameters of the relationship prior to providing their consent. In the context of both psychotherapy and gaming, informed consent should occur as early as possible. From an ethical perspective, informed consent serves as a keystone of professional practice, ensuring that practitioners adhere to their profession's code of ethics and that clients obtain the necessary information to make rational choices about their treatment (Fallon, 2006). The informed consent process should be collaborative in nature and set clear expectations. Though the exact topics covered may change depending on the provider's license and location of practice, several topics should be universally covered. Such topics include privacy policies and limitations to confidentiality (i.e., mandatory and permissive reporting, as well as the limitations inherent in group therapy), potential risks, alternative treatments, the voluntary nature of participation, expectations regarding client and therapist roles, group rules and norms, group duration, payment, and session content (e.g., subject matter and narrative themes; APA, 2017). When routine outcome monitoring (ROM) measures are utilized to track client progress over time, informed consent regarding how the data will be collected and used must be obtained from clients or their parent.

All participants should have a clear understanding of what to expect from groups prior to joining. At times, parents of youth participants may be tempted to tell their participants that the TA-RPG group they are joining is "just fun." While it may not be appropriate to delve into treatment goals with these participants, parents should be guided to be candid about the general goals of the group—for social flourishing TA-RPG groups, this often includes engaging in a safe space to collaborate with other people, create a shared story, and increase social confidence through engagement in a fun activity.

Group and Setting Considerations

Size

Group size varies based on the needs of the client, facilitator, and setting. However, the recommended group size is four to six participants in order to ensure each individual has adequate and balanced opportunities to fully engage each session. Though groups of seven or more participants are possible, a large number of players can be unwieldy and may result in diminishing returns for individual growth and participation.

Routine Outcome Monitoring

ROM has been shown to improve treatment outcomes and can act as an early warning sign in treatment for client unresponsiveness or deterioration (Boswell et al., 2015). Additionally, ROM can be useful in better understanding the efficacy of treatment and change processes in psychotherapy (Gondek et al., 2016). Practices and organizations that already use standardized measures should continue to use them across TA-RPG groups. When ROM measures are unavailable, feedback from clients as well as parents (if applicable) should be regularly solicited throughout treatment. Such feedback allows therapists to adjust therapeutic interventions and story content to better fit the needs of clients.

Parent Feedback and Participation

Full engagement in TA-RPG groups requires vulnerability and trust. Due to the nature of such interventions, non-group members (e.g., parents, spouses, friends) should not be permitted to observe or participate in the group under normal circumstances. As an alternative, it is recommended that TA-RPG facilitators educate clients and parents regarding treatment expectations (e.g., a typical session outline) and be prepared to provide a plan and rationale for linking treatment goals to in-game content. Additionally, parents may benefit from education focusing on effective ways to talk to their children about their sessions and progress. Parents can be supported to inquire about narrative content, convey interest in their child's character, and ask broad questions such as "how did the group work together?" Conversely, questions such as "what did you learn?" or "what skills (goals) did you work on?" may be inappropriate for children who are uninterested in or unaware of the therapeutic processes of their treatment. Although straightforward questions may be appropriate for participants with concrete goals, a significant portion of the therapeutic intervention within TA-RPG occurs during gameplay and is covert. As a result, change processes may not be immediately apparent to children and adolescents. Overall, parents' questions regarding the skills and insights their children have gained are often effectively answered through inquiry into the game's narrative and the child's experience.

In addition to providing education around client–parent communication, facilitators should schedule periodic meetings with parents. Meetings such as these serve as opportunities to review treatment goals and gauge progress since the initial screening session. Additionally, providers should elicit feedback from parents about changes they have noticed in the client (i.e., at home and school) and about the client's experience in the group. Finally, provider–parent meetings can help to identify new goals and to address any questions, comments, or concerns related to treatment.

Homework

TA-RPGs are generally designed as an in-session intervention, without explicit between-session work. However, for some groups and individuals, between-session engagement in TA-RPG-related activities may serve to support their goals. When used appropriately, homework can serve as an effective and pragmatic tool for expanding treatment beyond the therapy room and enhancing treatment outcomes. When treatment goals include community reintegration or engagement in new hobbies, and the client is amenable, homework can be assigned as an additional component of treatment. Such an addition serves as a transitional bridge from TA-RPG to recreational TTRPG games online and in their community.

Following is a list of homework assignments that have been used in TA-RPG groups. Although some assignments presented here are free, several require an entrance fee, purchasing supplies, access to the Internet, or travel. The feasibility and rationale of assignments should be discussed with clients and/or parents in advance to increase engagement. When appropriate, completion of assignments can be tied to in-game rewards, such as obtaining magical objects, gold, or credit toward leveling up their characters. It is important to be careful about leveraging these in-game rewards too strongly, as it may adversely impact the intrinsic rewards present in TA-RPG.

1. Look up game stores in your area.
2. Visit a game store.
3. Visit a game store to learn about opportunities for RPG activities (e.g., playing, crafting).
4. Attend a store-run or online RPG session.
5. Draw/paint/illustrate your character.
6. Purchase and paint a mini of your character.
7. Come up with a story about something your character is proud of.
8. Write a story about something your character is ashamed of.
9. Create a new character you would like to play.
10. Create an NPC.

Materials

TA-RPG groups can be run with minimal equipment, which can increase the ease of introducing them in settings that may be resistant to a new modality or have limited resources for interventions. The TA-RPG facilitator will need to confirm they have the materials necessary to begin their group. Following is a list of the general requirements, as well as different ways to fulfill each.

- Game System
- Randomizing Agent
- Game Tokens, Maps, etc.
- Character Sheets

Game System

The game system is the set of rules, guidelines, and general expectations for play. The game system will guide character creation and world building, and will set up the mechanics for how players and game masters (GMs) navigate social, exploration, and combat encounters. Usually a game system has a document or book containing the basic rules needed to play such as the Player's Handbook in Dungeons & Dragons, or a set of starting materials necessary to play such as the materials provided in Critical Core. Choosing a system is discussed further in Chapter 6.

Randomizing Agents

TTRPG systems frequently use a randomizing agent, the specifics of which are determined by the game system being used. In addition to character skills, these randomizing agents determine the outcome of events in the game and are crucial to play. For dice-based systems, physical dice and virtual dice can both be used, though physical dice may be especially appropriate for in-person games. The facilitator may benefit from providing a set of dice for each participant to use, though some participants may want to acquire and use their own set of dice. While it may be possible to use a single set of dice for the entire group to use or have players share dice, the frequency that players will need to simultaneously roll dice will likely result in a slower game.

When physical dice are not appropriate or available, there are a multitude of virtual options. Search engines and mobile device applications can be used to generate random numbers. Many voice-controlled intelligent personal assistant devices or smart speakers can roll dice with commands like "Roll a d20," and are accessibility supports for players who may not be able to otherwise roll physical dice. Many online TTRPG platforms have built-in rolling capabilities that will also add relevant bonuses and provide a final result without requiring the player to do any math.

When beginning a group and choosing the right type of dice to use, the facilitator should consider the needs and preferences of the group. Physical dice offer an enjoyable tactile sensation for players, which can further encourage engagement in the game and the hobby.

In virtual groups, physical dice rolls that are reported verbally to the GM require a level of trust that the results are reported honestly. As many virtual dice rollers have the capacity to share results with the group instantly, rolling virtual dice together online may increase the feelings of cohesion and excitement for other's dice rolls while reducing the pressure and ability to lie about physical dice rolls.

Game Tokens, Maps, etc.

TTRPGs can be played almost completely in the group's imagination, often taking place in person around a table or through a virtual video call. However, it can sometimes be helpful to have some physical representations and visualizations through the use of maps and images of key places and characters. For groups that connect virtually, there are multiple online platforms (both free and for a cost) that support the inclusion of maps and images, and can allow players to move the virtual tokens representing their characters. Groups that meet in person can utilize a whiteboard or wet-erase grid with tokens or miniatures as these representations. Facilitators running groups in person should also have some kind of barrier between the players and their notes and dice rolls, often called a "GM screen." This can allow the GM to keep notes hidden from the characters such as story directions and monster attributes, as well as reminders of system rules and mechanics.

Character Sheets

When starting a group, TA-RPG facilitators will determine whether they will use pre-made character sheets or have players create original characters. Both options have benefits and drawbacks. It can be valuable for the TA-RPG provider to collaborate with the client to create a custom character from scratch. This is most readily accomplished individually during the screening session or as a group during the first session. Individuals who are less experienced with a particular TTRPG ruleset for character creation, or individuals with limited time, may find third-party applications (e.g., D&D Beyond) to be a useful tool for both creating and updating characters. Many virtual character sheet management systems also provide additional information about skills, spells, and abilities by clicking on the element. This can support player autonomy and ownership over the character, as well as reduce the time in session spent looking up or discussing abilities. In some cases, the full character creation process cannot be completed in a single session. However, having the client identify and express their basic conceptualization of their character typically provides enough information to translate the idea into a character sheet outside of session, either by the participant or by the facilitator.

Custom character creation can be an arduous process, depending on the game system being played, and therefore can be unfeasible or unnecessary in some settings. Many TTRPG system publishers provide pre-made character sheets for free online. When utilizing pre-made sheets, we recommended they remain as customizable as possible. For example, omitting certain character details, such as name, alignment, physical characteristics, mobility or other assistive devices used, personality traits, and backstory information, can allow clients to maintain agency over the "flavor" of their character, without requiring clients to understand the game mechanics associated with character creation. Further, similar to custom characters, pre-made character options also provide opportunities for creativity. For example, clients may be encouraged to create detailed backstories for their characters, or to design portraits, crests, or other details that can be added to their character sheets. When using pre-made character sheets, it is important that a range of character types are given for participants to choose from.

Character sheets will be continuously updated as characters gain abilities, learn more about their background or skills, and use, trade, and receive items. In in-person groups, facilitators should consider keeping the player's character sheets between sessions, to prevent them from getting lost. Virtual character sheets stored in an online drive or a character management system can be an excellent way to provide players access to character sheets during online sessions or between sessions.

Modules

While each session should be prepared with intentionality, aligned with the individual and group needs, it may help TA-RPG facilitators to have an adventure module prepared in advance. Facilitators can create their own adventure module (potentially using the techniques for collaborative campaign creation in Chapter 11) or they can acquire pre-written adventure modules from other sources. For more information on pre-written adventure modules, see Chapter 7.

Online TA-RPG

Most of this book assumes in-person groups in which players are meeting with the GM in a shared physical space where the group is seated around a table. It is worth noting, however, that a tremendous value can be obtained through facilitating TA-RPG groups through online video conferencing platforms. Facilitating TA-RPG online provides access to the modality for individuals who may otherwise struggle to participate for a variety of reasons.

For many participants, the online medium will prioritize their health and safety. In the advent of the COVID-19 pandemic, it became safer to facilitate groups virtually than for clients to continue to meet in person for TA-RPG services. Virtual meetings allowed for a continuity of programming without interruption, while allowing for individuals to meet their needs and comfort level with potential contagion. Likewise, individual participants in hospital/medical settings are able to participate in virtual groups who would otherwise be unable to meet in person.

In addition to meeting health and safety needs around avoiding in-person contact, virtual groups are better suited to the accessibility needs of some players. Meeting virtually allows players to easily leverage a multitude of accessibility supports that may otherwise be difficult to integrate into an in-person TA-RPG program. Because virtual groups are implemented through computers, tablets, smartphones, or other electronic devices, integration of accessibility tools such as screen readers, text-to-speech, and magnification are seamless.

Virtual groups provide some individuals access to TA-RPG that may otherwise be impossible. Because TA-RPG is a rare intervention, individuals living at distances from TA-RPG facilitators are able to access services that would have otherwise been impossible. Traveling to meet in-person groups may be difficult for some participants because of travel and mobility challenges (e.g., a parent who is unable to drive a participant to the session because of a conflicting work schedule). Virtual programs allow for participants to meet from the convenience of their home.

The increased geographic area accessible by virtual TA-RPG groups also allows for facilitators to recruit from larger populations of participants. The facilitator can intentionally construct cohorts of participants with similar or complementary goals. Special interest groups may be difficult to assemble when limited by geographic region and access to transportation, but virtual groups remove barriers that enable construction of meaningful ensembles.

When beginning virtual programs, facilitators must consider additional factors, such as which conferencing platform to use, their own and their participants' technological needs, and how they will adapt physical aspects of TTRPGs to the virtual context (e.g., dice, character sheets, battle maps). The facilitator must choose and become proficient in the video conferencing platform they choose and be able to support participants in learning to use it. They must decide whether players will use physical dice and report results to the GM or whether the group will use an electronic dice-rolling system that shows results through the shared platform. Similarly, in-person TA-RPG groups feature character sheets printed on paper. Virtual groups may require access to electronic character sheets, or the facilitator may request participants print their own character sheets to have it physically in their own space. These conversations must be had with participants in an intake process, and the facilitator must be prepared to troubleshoot and problem-solve these issues regularly.

Virtual groups provide additional tools that may enhance the TA-RPG experience. Online tools such as virtual whiteboards allow for collaborative drawing or brainstorming, and many video conferencing platforms feature the ability to share videos, images, or sounds to increase immersion and player engagement. Additional communication tools, such as direct messages, allow the GM and players to communicate directly in ways that would be difficult in person, allowing for confidential communication of sensitive topics in a group setting, as well as sharing directly with the facilitator any discomfort with content or story elements.

Finally, virtual groups provide additional challenges that the facilitator must be prepared to navigate. The technological requirements for video conferencing may strain the resources of some participants. They may not have sufficient Internet speed at their home, or have camera and microphone equipment that make communication challenging (e.g., reverb on a microphone or a pixelated camera). Similarly, some participants may only have one location from which they can join virtually, which may be a central room in their home. This may mean that there will be background noise as well as confidentiality concerns that must be navigated by the group.

Session Zero/Session One

"Session zero" is the term commonly used in TTRPG groups to refer to a pre-gameplay session in which players engage as a group in an informed consent process. This often includes group agreements about logistics such as scheduling as well as group expectations around play style, story content, and safety tools. Because of the complex experiential nature of the game, it may not be possible to have a comprehensive session zero with a player who has never played a TTRPG before. Additionally, session zeros oriented toward background and logistics around a game with which they are unfamiliar may be boring. Implementing a session zero with new players, especially ambivalent or resistant participants, may reduce their buy-in and willingness to participate. For new groups, it is recommended to start with a session one that includes elements of a traditional session zero, such as the introduction of safety tools. Many of the other topics introduced in session zero (i.e., informed consent, topics to be avoided, time and meeting expectations) should have been addressed in the intake and informed consent process.

Here is a sample outline of a session one for a social flourishing group:

1. Introductions
2. Check-In Question (introduction of and participation in ritual)
3. Brief outline of safety tools including no/please list
4. Character choice (picking from pre-made characters)
5. Game play
6. Check out questions (spotlight, challenge, prediction)
7. Review of game play/notes about changing characters or questions

Here is a sample outline of a session one for a counseling group:

1. Introductions
2. Check-In Question (introduction of and participation in ritual)
3. Brief outline of safety tools including no/please list
4. Character choice (picking from pre-made characters)
5. Game play
6. Check out questions (spotlight, challenge, prediction)
7. Processing
8. Review of game play/notes about changing characters or questions

These structures should be adapted to the needs of individual settings and participants. The key components of the first session are the establishment of rituals such as the check-in and check-out structures, identification of characters, introduction of safety tools, and experience of game play. For the first session, a relatively straightforward and universally interesting story hook should be utilized. Additionally, even if potential triggers have been previously identified to the facilitator, a conservative approach to content should be utilized, and the facilitator should avoid commonly triggering material (i.e., graphic violence, intimate partner violence and sexual assault, spiders and other common phobias). Group norms will change as the group continues to develop, and it is often valuable to have some gameplay and experience (one to two sessions) with the group before developing more explicit table expectations, especially as this can create space for this discussion to be more participant-led, and it breaks up the "administrative" conversations across sessions.

Safety Tools

There are multiple types of safety tools that have been designed for in-person and virtual TTRPG groups. Two such tools are highlighted here, and facilitators must identify those that are the best fit for their particular populations and setting.

No/Please List

This safety tool is a twist on the common Yes/No list used in TTRPGs. The "no" list refers to potentially triggering content, typically explained to clients as content that would make them feel unsafe or uncomfortable in the group. This list should include trauma-related triggers, as well as other content that may make the player so uncomfortable that it would interfere with their participation in the group. Common "no" list topics include torture, sexual assault, spiders, sexual content, and racism and other forms of bigotry. With topics related to discrimination, it may be helpful to clarify with the participant if they would like none of this in the world of the story (i.e., a world without sexism), or if they would like it to exist in the world, but have it not directed at them. Some participants want discrimination to exist in such a fantasy setting where they may have more power to address and challenge such discrimination.

In addition to participant "no" lists, facilitators should have their own "no" list. This list should include topics that would be inappropriate for the group and setting, as well as items that the facilitator has personal boundaries around. Though some of these items may not be listed publicly (i.e., "sexually explicit content" may not be listed on the public "no" list, but would be inappropriate for a young adolescent group), identification of one or two of the facilitator's "no" items can be a valuable way for the facilitator to model setting a boundary.

The "please" list is a list of things players would like to request in the game. The "please" title as opposed to the "yes" title helps to clarify that this is a list of hopes, not expectations. Players may choose to request story content (e.g., a battle between lycanthropes and vampires), thematic content (e.g., political intrigue and subterfuge), as well as requests for specific in-game representation (e.g., matriarchal societies instead of European-inspired patriarchies and inclusion of non-heterosexual relationships). The "please" list is an open-ended invitation for players to share with the facilitator the kind of experience they would like to have in the TTRPG and an opportunity for the GM to model a willingness to listen and consider the requests of the players.

Both lists should be given privately to the facilitator. They may be shared directly with a facilitator during an intake or screening session. During an in-person group, they may be written by participants on index cards and passed face-down to the facilitator. In a virtual meeting, they may be shared through a private chat or online form submission. Once the facilitator has lists from all participants, they can be combined and presented to the group as a whole. This allows for the participants to be aware of the complete "no" and "please" lists, but keeps the identity of who added each item private. Participants should be invited to update these lists as they gain more experience with the group and the game.

There may be times that players include items on their "no" list that may require follow-up conversation either individually or as a group. A "no" list item may prompt follow-up or inquiry in individual counseling if it indicates a concern (i.e., a very specific example of child abuse). Similarly, if a participant adds something to their "no" list that may be inappropriate for other participants (i.e., a teen making a very specific and explicit reference to a sexual subculture in their "no" list), it will be important that the facilitator not inadvertently expose the other participants to the inappropriate content.

If a participant adds discriminatory content to their "no" list (i.e., a request to have no gay characters), the facilitator may choose to engage with the participant individually or in a group discussion, depending on the group and the individual's goals, as well as the facilitator's training and capacity to navigate the situation. It may be a worthwhile opportunity for exploring openness to others, understanding one's individual biases, as well as to engage in values clarification.

Pausing Gameplay

There may be times in the middle of a game session, even in the middle of high-intensity role-play, that a facilitator will need to pause the game and check in with the participants. This can be confusing for participants if the GM is role-playing a non-player character (NPC) and must suddenly shift into a facilitator role to address a concern. Similarly, because not every GM or player will portray characters with a clear voice or embodiment, it may be unclear when someone is speaking as themselves or as a character, and interactions may be taken personally and feelings hurt as a result. If the GM has a shorthand word or phrase, possibly including a physical gesture, to indicate a pause in the story, the game can quickly and efficiently be interrupted and resumed. One such technique, "zipping out," is particularly useful with youth participants. When the GM is interrupting the play, they will hold up a hand and mime pulling down a zipper, almost as if opening the entrance to a tent. With the word "Zip!" they indicate to the players that the simulation is paused and the players can interact as themselves, during which an issue can be addressed and resolved. When the game is to be resumed, the facilitator uses the same word "Zip!" and mimes zipping the zipper back up.

For adult participants or those who may balk at the silliness of a facilitator unzipping the barrier between reality and fiction, a similar phrase and analogous gesture may likewise be helpful. A GM or other participant can put their hand flat on the top of their head, or hold up their hands in a "T" shape (gestures likely not performed regularly) to indicate that they are speaking out of character to another participant or to the GM. The inclusion of the verbal signal "pause" may be additionally helpful. The specific word or phrase and gesture will be determined by the facilitator depending on their own comfort and in accordance with the group's needs.

Confidentiality/Outside of Group Contact

For many social flourishing groups, outside of group contact is both encouraged and a great sign of progress. However, not all groups, populations, or settings are appropriate for participants to communicate outside of the group. In settings in which outside of group contact is allowed, and such behavior is not clinically contraindicated or otherwise inappropriate, expectations about such contact and potential implications should be discussed with group members as part of an informed consent process about such behavior. Typically this conversation invites the participants to consider the pros and cons of spending time with each other outside of the group. It can be exciting for participants to spend time with people with shared interests that they have had positive experiences with in the group. However, the group is a special kind of setting, with a facilitator to support communication. The group or dyad dynamics may look different outside of such a supportive environment. Additionally, if there is out-of-group conflict that impacts in-group play, participants must be willing to address that conflict in group if needed. Many groups will want to play with and support each other outside of the group setting, while other groups will prefer to keep their relationship confined to the group space during the course of the group.

References

American Psychological Association. (2017). *Ethical principles of psychologists and code of conduct (2002, amended effective June 1, 2010, and January 1, 2017)*. Retrieved from www.apa.org/ethics/code/

Arenas, D. L., Viduani, A., & Araujo, R. B. (2022). Therapeutic use of role-playing game (RPG) in mental health: A scoping review. *Simulation & Gaming, 53*(3), 285–311. https://doi.org/10.1177/10468781211073720

Bernard, H., Burlingame, G., Flores, P., Greene, L., Joyce, A., Kobos, J. C., ... & Feirman, D. (2008). Clinical practice guidelines for group psychotherapy. *International Journal of Group Psychotherapy, 58*(4), 455–542. https://doi.org/10.1521/ijgp.2008.58.4.455

Boswell, J. F., Kraus, D. R., Miller, S. D., & Lambert, M. J. (2015). Implementing routine outcome monitoring in clinical practice: Benefits, challenges, and solutions. *Psychotherapy Research, 25*(1), 6–19. https://doi.org/10.1080/10503307.2013.817696

Burlingame, G. M., McClendon, D. T., & Alonso, J. (2011). Cohesion in group therapy. *Psychotherapy, 48*(1), 34–42. https://doi.org/10.1037/a0022063

Fallon, A. (2006). Informed consent in the practice of group psychotherapy. *International Journal of Group Psychotherapy, 56*(4), 431–453. https://doi.org/10.1521/ijgp.2006.56.4.431

Frances, A., Clarkin, J. F., & Marachi, J. P. (1980). Selection criteria for outpatient group psychotherapy. *Psychiatric Services, 31*(4), 245–250. https://doi.org/10.1176/ps.31.4.245

Gondek, D., Edbrooke-Childs, J., Fink, E., Deighton, J., & Wolpert, M. (2016). Feedback from outcome measures and treatment effectiveness, treatment efficiency, and collaborative practice: A systematic review. *Administration and Policy in Mental Health and Mental Health Services Research, 43*(3), 325–343. https://doi.org/10.1007/s10488-015-0710-5

Greenberg, R. P., Constantino, M. J., & Bruce, N. (2006). Are patient expectations still relevant for psychotherapy process and outcome? *Clinical Psychology Review, 26*(6), 657–678. https://doi.org/10.1016/j.cpr.2005.03.002

Henrich, S., & Worthington, R. (2021). Let your clients fight dragons: A Rapid Evidence Assessment regarding the therapeutic utility of 'Dungeons & Dragons'. *Journal of Creativity in Mental Health*, 1–19. https://doi.org/10.1080/15401383.2021.1987367

Kilmer, J., & Kilmer, E. D. (2018, July). *Therapeutic benefits of role-playing games* [Address]. Waco VA Community Mental Health Summit, Waco, TX.

Ragins, B. R., & Ehrhardt, K. (2021). Gaining perspective: The impact of close cross-race friendships on diversity training and education. *Journal of Applied Psychology, 106*(6), 856–881. https://doi.org/10.1037/apl0000807

Stone, D. M., Holland, K. M., Bartholow, B., Crosby, A. E., Davis, S., & Wilkins, N. (2017). *Preventing suicide: A technical package of policies, programs, and practices*. National Center for Injury Prevention and Control, Centers for Disease Control and Prevention. Retrieved from www.cdc.gov/violenceprevention/pdf/suicideTechnicalPackage.pdf

Substance Abuse and Mental Health Services Administration (SAMHSA). (2020). *Treatment for suicidal ideation, self-harm, and suicide attempts among youth*. Retrieved from https://store.samhsa.gov/sites/default/files/SAMHSA_Digital_Download/PEP20-06-01-002.pdf

Weiler, L. M., Helfrich, C. M., Palermo, F., & Zimmerman, T. S. (2013). Exploring diversity attitudes of youth placed in residential treatment facilities. *Residential Treatment For Children & Youth, 30*(1), 23–39. https://doi.org/10.1080/0886571X.2013.751790

Yalom, I., & Leszcz, M. (2020). *Theory and practice of group psychotherapy* (6th ed.). Basic Books.

14

Spreading the Word

Sharing the Magic of Therapeutically Applied Role-Playing Games

At this stage in the book, therapeutic game masters (GMs) should have the foundational knowledge required to implement therapeutically applied role playing game (TA-RPG) groups with populations they are competent to work with. However, to effectively start and run a TA-RPG group, facilitators must also have skills and knowledge to communicate about TA-RPG groups with group stakeholders and potential referral sources about the utility of TA-RPGs. This may include conversations with administrators, other clinicians, educators, community groups, parents, and potential participants. This chapter will cover recommendations around communicating about the use of TA-RPGs: Getting fellow clinicians and administrators on board, developing a referral network, communicating with potential participants, and addressing common misconceptions about tabletop role-playing games (TTRPGs).

Know *Your* Group

As discussed throughout this book, TA-RPGs can be an appropriate intervention for a wide range of individuals with many different presenting concerns and goals. However, each individual group will have a narrower range of demographics, problems, and goals appropriate for the group. Facilitators are encouraged to identify characteristics of ideal participants for their groups. When communicating with potential clients or referral sources, inclusion and exclusion criteria for the group should be clearly outlined.

When speaking with a potential referral source, it can be tempting for facilitators to describe their groups as open and accessible to everyone. While the creation of a safe and welcoming environment is essential to group success, TA-RPG groups generally have inclusion and exclusion criteria aligned with the intended function of the group (i.e., a group for adolescent girls who experience social anxiety, or a group for veterans who want to improve communication skills). Expressing that a group is open to anyone not only means that the facilitator may get referrals that

DOI: 10.4324/9781003281962-14

end up being a poor fit for the group, but also means that it is unlikely to stay in the mind of the therapist, teacher, or medical provider who might otherwise refer a participant to the group.

When providing a referral, the referring professional will typically meet a client or student, find out their challenges or goals, and then provide suitable resources that they think would be a good fit for their needs. As a result, if the group is explained to the referring professional as open to everyone, then they may not think of it as a service when the right client comes along. If the ideal candidate for the group is a participant between the ages of 13 and 15 with challenges related to neurodiversity and exploring gender identity, then sharing that specific information with referral sources is far more likely to make for a successful referral.

Develop a Pitch

A pitch is a quick and easy to understand description of services that can be verbally described to someone. Facilitators should develop and practice a clear and concise description of their services, highlighting their benefits and the kinds of individuals who might utilize them.

On the basis of the authors' experience, we recommend that facilitators start by developing three pitches: A "single breath" pitch, which is no more than one or two sentences in length, an "elevator" pitch, which is 30 seconds or less in length, and an "interested" pitch, which is a more full description of services and benefits up to five minutes in length. Additionally, the facilitator should be able to deliver the single breath pitch and the elevator pitch without needing to mention the specific game, or any descriptions of game mechanics, being used in the TTRPG group. Practicing a pitch for individuals who have little to no experience with TTRPGs, as well as those who are experienced, can be helpful. Facilitators should be practiced enough with their pitch to adjust the language based on the needs and knowledge of the individuals to whom they will most likely be pitching.

Know Your Audience

When two of the authors of this book, Adam D. Davis and Adam R. Johns, were initially expanding their TA-RPG groups, they had the opportunity to speak at a parent–teacher association (PTA) meeting at a local middle school. Excited to share the life-enriching opportunities TA-RPGs have to offer, they regaled the audience with tales of collaborative adventures through magical lands. As TA-RPG facilitators, they clearly saw the narratives of growth, insight, and change in the stories they told. However, the PTA members did not have the background understanding of TTRPGs, did not hear information that was relevant to their needs, and did not have the time, energy, or interest to ask clarifying follow-up questions. As a result, Johns and Davis were given a cold send-off from the principal and lost the opportunity to serve the students at the school. Instead of leading with their enthusiasm, describing epic moments fighting dragons, they should have expressed what the educators would have found relevant to their needs: The groups were aimed at improving students' frustration tolerance, helping them work in groups, and building their communication skills. The teachers likely would have wanted to know how TA-RPG groups would support classroom learning, and the principal would have been intrigued by the concept that TA-RPG groups may result in a reduction of behavior outbursts and disciplinary office referrals. Their presentation to the PTA was filled with specific terms from the game and moments of player character success, but lacked the details of most interest to their audience. They learned this lesson early in their careers so that future facilitators do not have to make the same mistake!

When recruiting for, and communicating about, TA-RPG groups, facilitators will need to identify multiple ways of describing the experiences and outcomes of their group in order to adjust their language to be accessible to their audience, and speak to their needs. A group of gamers familiar with TTRPGs might want to know that the group uses Dungeons & Dragons (D&D) with good-aligned player characters, and focuses on a collaborative homebrew world. A group of parents unfamiliar with TTRPGs would need to know that it is a game played mostly with imagination where the players work on a team and build strong positive social connections with one another. An administrator may want to understand the cost of implementation, other locations where it has been successful, or the potential risks for clients. All of these descriptions are true, each one adjusted to be more likely to resonate with the knowledge and needs of the audience. When possible, it can be extremely helpful for facilitators to meet with a sample of their potential audience to ask questions about the information and outcomes that these individuals are most interested in hearing about, and use that information to shape introductory pitches and marketing materials.

Pitching to a Supervisor

Some facilitators are passionate about the idea of getting their own TA-RPG group started within a setting that requires approval of a supervisor or manager. Facilitators who have a supervisor who is already aware of the benefits and growth potential of TA-RPGs may not need to prepare any more than they would for any other meeting. For facilitators with supervisors unfamiliar with the intervention, it can be helpful to have a few talking points which are prepared in advance and available to use to help educate the supervisor and address any potential concerns.

Activity Description

Facilitators should develop a clear, concise, and straightforward description of the group experiences that does not rely on any knowledge of the game on the part of the listener. It can be helpful to assume that the supervisor has already been misinformed about how TTRPGs are played, and be ready with nonjudgmental corrective information.

Facilitators should aim to include the following information in a quick activity description:

- The activity is not a video game.
- The participants play on a team together, rather than competitively.
- The game is played with descriptions and imagination.
- Because the intervention does not "feel" like traditional therapeutic interventions, it can be a particularly good fit for participants uninterested in or fatigued from more traditional interventions.
- The goal of the game is for the participants and facilitator to collaboratively create a story together.

Facilitators may also include a short story about an in-game encounter with a clearly articulated moment of growth. To prevent unintentional reinforcement of common misunderstandings about TTRPGs, facilitators should generally avoid the following topics in initial short pitches.

- The name of the TTRPG.
- Any words referring to the combat of the game (i.e., combat, death, battle, swords, killing).
- Any specific description of the rules of the game, including what dice to roll or what attributes or bonuses characters may have.
- Stories about what happens in the game that are rambling and/or do not clearly articulate a point of growth to the listener.

If the facilitator has the opportunity for a longer pitch, or the supervisor expresses interest or questions, these topics should be discussed. When providing this information, opportunities for questions and discussion about common misconceptions can be helpful in ensuring the supervisor understands the content. Facilitators should not lie about the experiences within the game or the aspects of play, but as this approach is still building in popularity, it is best to present the most relevant and applicable information first.

Benefits and Outcomes

Facilitators should have a clear statement of the benefits that TTRPGs could bring to this particular population. Examples may be pulled from other locations within this text, but a good starting point is the Core Capacities, discussed in Chapter 8.

Supporting Research

Having a set of research which helps to support the establishment of TA-RPG groups can be very helpful. We encourage all facilitators to continue to stay informed of the latest research related to this field, especially as it is an emerging specialty, and newly released research is still highly impactful to the field. Facilitators can find research information on the Game to Grow website at www.gametogrow.org, as well as throughout this text. Being prepared with this research will help lend support to a supervisor pitch, and will demonstrate a strong knowledge of the subject matter.

Available TA-RPG Resources

Some supervisors will want to know that the facilitator has adequate training in the model of approach that they want to use, and that there are resources which can be used to help support their continued education. Game to Grow, along with several other organizations, offers training and ongoing consultations, which can help support facilitators with challenges that may come up within their group setting. It is strongly recommended to seek these additional training resources when starting a group for the first time.

Inexpensive Materials

Many supervisors must maintain a program budget and are often concerned about the cost of introducing new programs. TTRPGs are generally inexpensive, requiring only a single book and some printed character sheets. Assuring the supervisor of the relatively small budget, especially if the facilitator already owns some of the materials, may help alleviate some of their concerns.

Other Successful Groups

It can be reassuring to many supervisors that the facilitator is not the first person to conduct this kind of therapeutic group. Having many examples of other locations that are providing these kinds of services may help bolster and reinforce the facilitator's claims. Facilitators can feel free to reference Game to Grow in this way.

Stay Open to Constructive Questions

Facilitators should understand that individuals who are unaware of TTRPGs may have questions about the experience, including questions which may seem obvious to a facilitator who has participated in the hobby for a long time. It is important that facilitators address these questions in a nonjudgmental way and are ready to clarify any misunderstandings surrounding TTRPGs, or their therapeutically applied counterpart.

Be Ethical

As with any intervention, it is important for facilitators to provide accurate information to their organization, referral sources, and potential clients. Facilitators should be clear about appropriate goals for their groups, and should never promise outcomes which are not supported by this intervention. Facilitators should always operate within the boundaries of their license and competency when providing TA-RPG services, just as they would with any other therapy services. Additionally, facilitators should use accurate language that the communities they work with will understand.

Connect With Providers With Complementary Skills

When developing a TA-RPG practice, much like any service, a trusted and informed referral network can be exceedingly beneficial. Facilitators who are working to build such a network should identify providers with complementary skill sets, such as family physicians, librarians, therapists, and after-school and peer-support facilitators. A healthy network of professionals and peers will bring in further referrals for services, as well as allow the facilitator to have a list of trusted sources of care which they can provide to participants and families as needed.

Educate Your Colleagues

For facilitators running groups within settings that utilize internal referral networks, such as hospitals, schools, or community mental health settings, educating fellow providers about TA-RPG groups can increase organizational buy-in and appropriate referrals. Facilitators should use techniques similar to the ones listed earlier to help their colleagues learn and know more about TA-RPGs.

When working in such settings, two of the authors, Jared N. and Elizabeth D. Kilmer, found success with a two-part method that is now utilized by Game to Grow to secure referrals from agencies, hospitals, and other organizations. First, they offered to provide a short lecture introduction to TA-RPGs as part of a lunch-and-learn or staff meeting. These presentations were tailored to the group in attendance (administrators, therapists, support staff, medical staff). Following the presentation, those who were interested were invited to attend a follow-up 30-minute workshop, in which attendees were able to interact with game materials and play through short encounters. During the play experience, attendees were encouraged to reflect on ways in which they believed an intervention using this game may be beneficial to their clients.

These educational experiences were not designed to train attendees in the use of TA-RPGs; they were designed to educate, inspire, and excite attendees about the potential uses with their clients and the wider population served. The authors found that attendees of these experiences were more likely to provide high-quality referrals, and often spontaneously provided information to other departments that could benefit from similar programming.

Addressing Common Misconceptions of TTRPGs

Though the popularity of TTRPGs has increased significantly in the last decade, there are still commonly held misconceptions, even among mental health professionals, that may create reluctance, confusion, or concern in stakeholders. In a study of psychiatrists, 22% of those surveyed reported a belief in a link between psychopathology and TTRPGs (Lis et al., 2015). If these misconceptions are not prevalent in the facilitator's community, it may not be necessary to include corrective information in promotional materials or introductory pitches; however, they should still feel comfortable addressing these concerns.

TTRPGs Are Video Games

Though this may be an especially prevalent misconception for virtually mediated TA-RPG groups, this confusion can occur even with in-person groups. Facilitators should clarify early, and sometimes often, that TTRPGs are a storytelling game played with descriptions and imagination, not a video game.

TTRPGs Are Only for Men/Adults/Children

Though some of the first editions of TTRPG systems used language that included only male players, individuals of all genders have a place in the TTRPG world (Garcia, 2017). In the last decades, the TTRPG community has become increasingly inclusive. While the idea of "game" may spark the concern that TTRPGs are "only for children," people of all ages can enjoy TTRPGs. We have had the opportunity to run TA-RPG groups for older adults who had no prior experience with fantasy and role-playing games. Many of those adults left their groups with newly identified hobbies in tabletop gaming. Facilitators can also speak to their own experiences with TTPRGs as well as those in their groups (both social and therapeutic).

TTRPGs Are Too Complicated

A common concern potential participants have is that they do not have enough experience with TTRPGs to join a TA-RPG group. For most TA-RPG groups, it is recommended that the facilitator have new participants playing the game within the first session, without the participant having any experience or prior knowledge of TTRPGs. In some cases, the participant may feel more comfortable joining a group if they are able to see examples of gameplay first. In these cases, the facilitator should be able to offer recommendations to a video or podcast that showcases play similar in genre to that of the TA-RPG group. In addition to offering this resource, the facilitator should set expectations regarding how the publicized gameplay and TA-RPG group's gameplay may look different.

TTRPGs Lead to Devil Worship

Depending on the setting and population, participants or other stakeholders may have concerns about the possible negative effects of engaging in TTRPGs. Many of these concerns stem from the "Satanic Panic" of the 1980s. It is important that TA-RPG providers have a basic understanding of the history and myths surrounding this event and can answer stakeholder questions and concerns.

In 1979, a private investigator who was hired to investigate the disappearance of a 16-year-old boy claimed that D&D was at the heart of the child's disappearance. Though the incident was later found to be unconnected to D&D or tabletop role-playing, the story was sensationalized and it sparked the novel and movie, *Mazes and Monsters* (Peterson, 2021). In 1982, following a high school student's death, his mother, Patricia Pulling, sued the school's principal (who ran her son's D&D games), as well as the company who created the game, before starting an organization called Bothered About Dungeons and Dragons (BADD). Though their cases were dismissed by the courts, she and her organization were part of a media campaign to discuss the perceived dangers of the game (BBC, 2014). Some conservative Christians, such as Jon Quigley (Lakeview Full

Gospel Fellowship), denounced the game as an "occult tool" that made young people vulnerable to "influence or possession by demons" (BBC, 2014). Evangelist Jack Chick created the comic Dark Dungeons to illustrate the supposed satanic nature of D&D (Riggs, 2016). Through the late seventies and early eighties, the combination of fear, ignorance surrounding the game, and norms within the gaming community, led to misinformation that proliferated and scared parents. One such myth was that if an individual's character died in game, the player would likely commit suicide (BBC, 2014). Other misunderstandings surrounded the fantasy element of the game—there were some thoughts that when players had their character cast a spell in the game, they were trying to cast the spell in real life (Riggs, 2016).

The concerns surrounding D&D were not dissimilar to those brought against other types of games and media with fantasy content. A fear that youth may struggle to tell the difference between fantasy and reality, as well as the belief that stories of magic and witchcraft were anti-biblical, contributed to apprehensions surrounding the game. It is important to note not all D&D settings and campaigns were appropriate for all ages. Many of the earlier books had risqué art or themes not appropriate for children (Peterson, 2021).

Since the late 1980s, the moral panic surrounding D&D and other TTRPGs has largely died down, and the games have continued to grow in popularity. They have been portrayed more positively in media, such as through representations in the popular TV shows "Stranger Things" and "Community," as well as the popular stream "Critical Role."

Conclusion

Therapeutically applied role-playing games are still an emerging approach, and as such may face more challenges than older, more established therapies. Being able to communicate this approach clearly and effectively with colleagues and potential new clients is important, not only for the success of each facilitator but also for the success of the field of TA-RPGs.

A Rising Tide Raises All Boats

The emerging field of TA-RPGs can be appealing and exciting for facilitators to dive into. At some point, facilitators may meet others, also jumping into this exciting field.

While we cannot tell you how to handle competition in your field, we can remind you that the field of TA-RPGs is wide open, and has plenty of space to expand. There is room for everyone who is excited to jump into this field. We hope that each new facilitator will help to welcome others into this field with the same welcoming attitude that we have brought to others, always remembering that a rising tide in the field of TA-RPGs raises all boats.

References

BBC. (2014, April 11). The great 1980s Dungeons & Dragons panic. *BBC News*. Retrieved July 24, 2021, from www.bbc.com/news/magazine-26328105

Garcia, A. (2017). Privilege, power, and Dungeons & Dragons: How systems shape racial and gender identities in tabletop role-playing games. *Mind, Culture, and Activity, 24*(3), 232–246. https://doi.org/10.1080/10749039.2017.1293691

Lis, E., Chiniara, C., Biskin, R., & Montoro, R. (2015). Psychiatrists' perceptions of role-playing games. *Psychiatric Quarterly, 86*(3), 381–384. http://doi.org/10.1007/s11126-015-9339-5

Peterson, J. (2021). *Game wizards: The epic battle for Dungeons & Dragons*. The MIT Press.

Riggs, B. (2016, April 13). How did gaming greats navigate the satanic panic of the 1980s? *Nerdist*. Retrieved July 24, 2021, from https://nerdist.com/article/how-did-gaming-greats-navigate-the-satanic-panic-of-the-1980s/

15

The Curse of the Viney Woods

An Example Module

No therapeutically applied role-playing game (TA-RPG) manual would be complete without an example module to jumpstart facilitators in the running of an effective session. The following module is designed to be applicable to a wide number of tabletop role-playing games (TTRPGs). This module has storylines, characters, game master (GM) guidance, and suggestions for how to enhance the therapeutic outcomes when it is being played. It does not contain any specific information about what rule to use, what dice to roll, or what kind of character class abilities the player characters may have.

This module is best suited for a GM style tabletop role-playing game that has a strategic ruleset, has players controlling a single character, and uses dice and attribute bonuses to determine success. Games that are a good fit for use with this module include Dungeons & Dragons, Pathfinder, and Critical Core. There are several references within the following modules to pages within Critical Core's materials which may help point to you a rule or statistic which may be helpful.

The format of this module is similar to the structure of a module in Critical Core. Each encounter is broken into sections providing instructions and helpful information for running the encounter. The storyline is designed to give the GM the right amount of information, without overwhelming newer GMs with too much information. Each encounter provides the necessary information to move the story forward, while leaving space for the facilitator to fill in the blanks with anything that may be helpful or needed for their players. The game sections are explained in the following.

Encounter Title

The title of the encounter gives you a small, flavorful, description to give you a brief idea of what the encounter is about. It also contains

DOI: 10.4324/9781003281962-15

some brief information of the type of encounter (i.e., Combat, Social, or Exploration), and a short summary of the Core Capacities which are most easily accessed for growth within this encounter.

Read-Aloud Script

This section is designed to be read out loud to the players and sets up the descriptions and obstacles in the way of the player characters. In most cases, this section should be read out loud as the first thing to happen within the encounter.

Game Master Summary

This section provides clear instructions for the GM about the challenges and information this encounter must contain including any important plot information that will need to be passed along to the players to keep the storyline together.

Desire

A short description of the player character's desire.

Obstacle

A short description of the obstacle in the way of the player character's achieving their desire.

Tactic

A short description of the likely tactics that will be employed by the player characters.

So Then

A section to be read out loud when the encounter has been completed. The So Then section is designed to lead directly into the Read-Aloud Script of the next encounter.

Desire, Obstacle, Tactic, and So Then are part of the DOTS system, described in greater detail in Chapter 10.

Game Master Notes

This section provides further suggestions and advice for how to enhance play and engagement within this story section. It includes advice for how to adjust this particular encounter, or broad advice for how to enhance the GM's skills in facilitating a great game.

Supporting Growth

This section details the Core Capacities (discussed in greater detail in Chapter 8), which are most accessible through this particular encounter, and provides suggestions for how to maximize those growth opportunities. It is important to keep in mind that player choices and facilitator responses may allow an encounter to highlight growth for an entirely different Core Capacity than the ones discussed in this section. The suggestions in this section are simply an option to further demonstrate and spotlight the areas of growth that this particular encounter may provide.

Encounter Outline

The heroes have been hired by the town of Wandershore to identify and remove a curse from the Viney Woods after some townspeople have gone missing after exploring that area. The town elder has provided the group with a map to the woods and their best guess as to the source of the disturbances.

The party crosses a rickety bridge and then meets a forest sprite who tells them that the disturbances are because of the vengeful ghost of an owlbear named Eera who was cruelly killed for sport and her body left in a cave to rot. The sprite tells them where they can find Eera's cave and how to put her to rest. The party is then attacked by wooden constructs that look like skeletons.

After the party defeats the skeletons and travels deeper into the woods, an unnatural frost rolls in. The party finds a cave entrance completely overgrown with vines that are frozen together. After they break through the frozen vines and travel deeper into the cave, they finally find the body of an owlbear, now long dead—the body of Eera. Before they can bury the body and say the burial incantation that the sprite taught them, the ghost of the owlbear appears and attacks them. They must defeat her, or talk her down, so that they can put her body to rest. In the epilogue, the heroes witness all of the villagers who had disappeared return to the village.

Table 15.1 The Six Encounters of The Curse of The Viney Woods

01	The Viney . . . Bridge?
The party must cross a rickety bridge that might not support their weight.	

02	Giggling Bushes
The party finds a forest sprite who provides more information about the quest, and a warning.	

03	Root of the Curse
Wooden skeletons attack, and the forest sprite shares how to break the curse.	

04	Frozen Vines
The party discovers a hidden cave, but frozen vines block the cave entrance.	

05	Burial rites
The heroes must quell Eera's ghost to perform the burial incantation and put her to rest.	

06	Epilogue
The heroes witness the vanished villagers return home and celebrate their accomplishment.	

Introduction Read-Aloud Script

"You have all been traveling together for some time as an adventuring team. Long enough that you know each other by name, and a little about your personalities. Long enough to know that you can trust your teammates to have your back.

You have been hired by a small town called Wandershore, off the coast of the Maraden sea. Wandershore does some fishing and small trade, but as you came into the town you found it to be largely unremarkable. However, upon hearing of some of your past jobs and heroic deeds, you were approached by the town eldar, a woman named Tensa.

Tensa explained that two men from the town, along with several strangers traveling with a caravan recently went missing while exploring the woods to the east. Tensa calles the area the Viney Woods, but it likely has several names depending on who you ask. Tensa claims that the Viney Woods have been cursed ever since she was a little girl, but the younger members of the town don't believe her.

Tensa has offered you each 15 gold [the game master can decide a different sum, if needed] *to find the source of the curse and break it. If possible, you're to find the missing townspeople and bring them back.*

After you accepted the quest from the town elder, Tensa, she drew you a basic map directing you toward the center of the Viney Woods."

Introduction Game Master Summary

This is a good opportunity for the GM to have the players introduce their characters and provide some details about their character's personality, background, or abilities. Some players may need more guidance on this than others, and may require some specific or pointed questions to elaborate on this character. Feel free to use the following list and select two to three questions that best fit your player's needs.

- What does your character look like? What are they wearing?
- Where is your character from? A big city or a small town?
- How did they decide to become an adventurer?
- Where did they learn their unique skills and abilities?
- What is something the other adventurers would have learned about your character through their travels together?
- What is something unique about your character?

Encounter 01: The Viney . . . Bridge?

The party must cross a ravine over a rickety bridge that might not support their weight.

Encounter Type: Exploration
Encounter Tone: Lighthearted
Core Capacities: Collaboration & Regulation

Read-Aloud Script

"As you follow the map that Tensa gave you, you're noticing a shift in the atmosphere of the forest itself. It is subtle, but it feels like the air is getting colder, even though it is midday, and the forest itself seems to be getting thinner and dryer. Almost like it is fall, when it is in fact the middle of summer.

> *Eventually you come to a wide clearing in the middle of the forest where there appears a large ravine. It cuts deep into the ground, at least 100 feet up or more, and you can see rushing water down below. The ravine stretches far to the north and south with no end in sight, but luckily there is a bridge made of wood and ropes that is stretching across the whole distance.*
>
> *Unfortunately, the bridge looks like it has gone a long time without any repair. You can see vines and plants growing along the distance, and many of the planks of wood have rotted out and fallen into the ravine. You're not certain that this bridge is safe, but it is currently your only way across."*

Game Master Summary

This is an exploration encounter with a very open-ended opportunity for collaborative problem solving.

The heroes must cross a rickety bridge over a ravine. This encounter is designed to allow the players some open-ended problem-solving possibilities (a quantum quandary, as described in Chapter 10).

As the players begin to cross the bridge, the GM can further describe and indicate that the bridge is unstable, potentially having pieces fall apart, or even the whole bridge crumble to pieces. The plot of this story assumes that the players will be successful in crossing the bridge and make it to the other side, so the GM should make sure that whatever tactics the players use results in this success.

The GM should provide opportunities with each attempt to make checks or have players roll dice. In general, ability checks should be a low difficulty level, and likely to succeed, but GMs should not let any one player solve the problem on their own, putting forward further obstacles or challenges related to crossing the bridge until every player has had an opportunity to help contribute to the solution.

The encounter ends when the players have made their way across the ravine and are ready to continue to follow the directions on the map. At that point read the "So Then" text.

Desire: Cross to the other side of the ravine.

Obstacle: The rickety bridge doesn't seem very stable.

Tactic: Traverse carefully, mend the bridge, find another way across.

So Then: *"Now safely on the other side of the ravine, you can continue to follow Tensa's map leading you deeper into the Viney Woods. Hopefully no more bridges await you."*

Game Master Notes

Running a successful quantum quandary can take some practice for new GMs, but when executed well, it can help all players feel a strong sense of autonomy within the game, and create a seamless collaborative storytelling experience.

In a quantum quandary each action that the player characters take provides a step toward the solution, even failed actions. When a player character is unsuccessful in their action (either it is impossible, or they are unsuccessful in their skill/attribute roll), the intent of their action should not succeed, but they may still uncover important information. For instance, a character may attempt to simply run quickly across the bridge. After a failed roll to determine their success, the GM describes that they get a running start, but then instantly fall through the first board that they step on. The player character doesn't fall into the ravine, instead catching themselves on the edge and pulling themselves back up. Even though they weren't successful, they uncovered important information, namely that the bridge planks are in worse shape than they originally thought, and cannot support their weight.

Supporting Growth

Core Capacities—Collaboration and Regulation

Because this is the first encounter in the module, players who have not played together before may be inclined to figure out a way for their individual character to cross the bridge (e.g., "My character will fly across"). However, the bridge is an excellent opportunity for players to experience the benefits of building on each other's ideas. To reinforce Collaboration in this encounter, the facilitator should be particularly responsive to player suggestions that include other players or build on their ideas, using their affect to show genuine interest and excitement about collaborative solutions. The GM can also spoon feed some collaboration ideas to help prompt collaborative thinking (e.g., "When you fly across, are you going to try to carry anyone else across with you?"). If a collaborative tactic is completely outlandish or the players have an unlucky roll of their dice, the facilitator can use the spectrum of yes (see Chapter 11) to move the heroes closer to their goal or provide an exciting result even if the tactic itself is not successful.

Not every character attempt will be successful, failed attempts are still an opportunity to build capacity for participants. High stakes situations are excellent for supporting the development of the Regulation capacity, as the failures create a sense of increased pressure. The facilitator should attune to the players responses, and can switch between participant and character pronouns and names to scaffold player Regulation (see Chapter 8). Helping players feel a sense of danger for their character, and then providing the tools and scaffolded support to regulate their emotions through that experience, will help them build those capacities in other portions of the game, as well as within their own lives.

Encounter 02: Giggling Bushes

The party finds a forest sprite who provides more information about the quest, and a warning.

Encounter Type: Social
Encounter Tone: Lighthearted
Core Capacities: Pretend Play, Perspective

Read-Aloud Script

"As you travel deeper into the Viney Woods, you can see why it has taken on that name. The trees all have a distinctive species of vine wrapping along the trunks, which seems to be stifling their growth. It creates an atmosphere of eerie death in a place that should teem with thriving life.

However, you've nearly reached the end of the map, and there doesn't appear to be anything of particular note within the woods around you. You'll need to find something to help point you in the direction of this curse.

As you are stepping through the woods, you suddenly hear a strange sound, like laughing coming from the bushes around you. The sound seems to shift from bush to bush at rapid speed, like an echo carrying on around you. In combination with the unusual woods, it creates an uneasy atmosphere, daring you to draw your weapon out."

Game Master Summary

This encounter is a role-play with a forest sprite named Kitcha. As she is native to the Viney Woods, she can pass through without being threatened. She is hesitant of the players, but is willing to get closer if they act friendly or seem to lower their guard.

Kitcha has important information, which must be shared with the group. It is detailed in the pop out section "Kitcha's Roleplay" in the next page.

No matter what tactic the players use, Kitcha will provide the information, as it is necessary to move the plot forward. Her demeanor will respond to player tactics, so she may be scared or friendly while providing it.

This encounter ends when the sprite has provided the necessary information. At that point, read the "so then" text, leading to the combat in the next encounter.

Desire: Get the forest sprite to share information about the woods.

Obstacle: The forest sprite is nervous, and she must be convinced to provide information.

Tactic: Stow weapons and show a friendly demeanor, or demand her assistance.

So Then: *"You have no idea how dangerous Eera can be," the sprite says to you in a frightened voice. As an unusual cold wind blows through the forest you can see her eyes widen and her ears perk up. "But I think you're about to find out." Before you can ask what that means, the forest sprite has vanished into the trees. You hear a whistling sound come from the woods"*

Role-playing Kitcha

Kitcha is a small forest sprite with humanoid features. She should be played as friendly but slightly nervous. If the players take aggressive action (or anything that might seem aggressive at first) have Kitcha clearly react strongly by diving back into the bushes out of reach. You can make Kitcha so extremely quick and dexterous that it is impossible for the players to catch her. If the players push the idea that they have to physically catch Kitcha, have her instead start talking to them from the bushes and trees, pushing the encounter into a dialogue instead of a chase or puzzle.

Kitcha needs to share the following information with the players. She can do so by simply offering it up to them, or you can work to engage the players in dialogue until they ask the right questions:

* The curse on the woods is caused by the vengeful spirit of an Owlbear named Eera, who was killed for sport and her body left to rot.
* The curse can be lifted if you find the body of the Owlbear and perform a burial ceremony on it, thanking it for its service to the woods.
* The body of Eera can be found in a cave to the east, with the entrance covered in vines.
* Eera's ghost is dangerous and vengeful, and has been capturing people who wander into the forest.
* Lastly, Kitcha will not travel with you deeper into the woods, it is not her job, but she will be appreciative of you being willing to remove the curse.

Game Master Notes

This is a good encounter for encouraging the players to use nonviolent tactics with NPCs. Kitcha may be playful, but will never attack or endanger the player characters. Have Kitcha demonstrate clear favoritism to any player who attempts a welcoming or friendly social tactic, providing that player with more time and attention for their attempts. Do not have players roll checks when using pro-social approaches, and instead let it be instantly successful.

If players attempt to attack Kitcha, you can have her escape or run back to the bushes and trees without allowing the player a dice roll to prevent it. Remember, you, the GM, always can decide that actions from the players can automatically succeed or fail without requiring a dice roll. This is a great space to be playful with players, using a different voice for Kitcha from the GM's usual speaking voice. Encourage the players to, also, speak as their characters using first person, and potentially also using a different sounding voice.

Supporting Growth

Core Capacity—Pretend Play

As this is the first role-play that the players have with an NPC, it will set a standard for future encounters and is a crucial opportunity to create an experience of pretend play. The facilitator should portray Kitcha with a personality different from their own. Many facilitators do this by changing their vocal quality (e.g., the speed, pitch) or by adjusting their body language to present themselves differently. When you, as the facilitator, can be playful and unembarrassed, you can help the players to feel safer and more welcome. Additionally, the pretend play demonstrated by Kitcha will help the players connect more readily with their own characters. Players may feel more comfortable easing into speaking in first person through their character, or providing their own character voice.

Encounter 03: Root of the Curse

Wooden skeletons attack, and the forest sprite shares how to break the curse.

Encounter Type: Combat
Encounter Tone: Serious
Core Capacities: Regulation, Planning

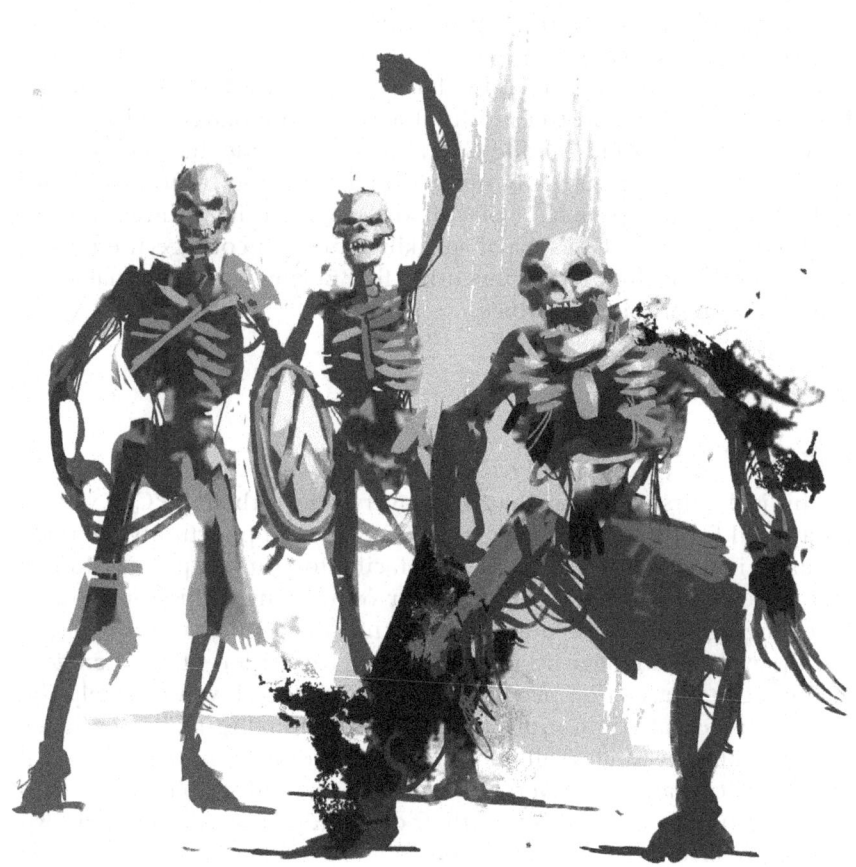

Figure 15.1 Wooden Skeletons

Read-Aloud Script

"*The whistling in the wind through the trees of the forest seems to hang in the air, getting louder and louder until it becomes much more of a screeching howl.*

From out of the surrounding forest you suddenly hear shuffling and groaning sounds, like wood being moved by strong winds. You see what look like humanoid skeletons, but clearly made of dried and dead wood shambling toward you (Figure 15.1). You're under attack, and you're surrounded. Defend yourself!"

Game Master Summary

> This is the first combat of this module, a fight with enemies that look like skeletons, but are actually made of wood.
>
> The wooden skeleton enemies are designed to be generally easy to face. GMs should make sure that the skeletons hit a couple of player characters once or twice so that they can feel like a threat, but this fight should be over in a couple of rounds.
>
> This encounter ends when the final skeleton is defeated.

Desire: Survive the attack from the skeletons.

Obstacle: The skeletons have sharp claws and won't allow the heroes to escape.

Tactic: Use weapons, spells, or other attacks to defeat the skeletons.

So Then: *"As the final skeletal facsimile falls to the ground you catch your breath and take a moment to gather yourself.*

[The player characters make take a break to recover if needed here]

Once you're ready, you begin to head to the east, toward the cave that Kitcha mentioned so that you can get rid of this curse once and for all."

Game Master Notes

Combat is a great way to help players feel like epic adventurers, and to bring them together as a team.

Reward teamwork-oriented actions by offering bonuses or advantages to help them be more successful.

Help encourage creativity from your players by allowing wacky or unusual ideas to be successful. This is a low-stakes combat, and the perfect place to let an unusual or goofy idea be successful, encouraging more creative thinking in the future.

Wooden Skeletons

GMs should prepare (or be ready to improvise) a monster or enemy statistics appropriate for these skeletons. GMs can adjust the monster to contain some special qualities listed here.

Special Qualities: Made of wood—While they look like skeletons, they are actually made of wood. The wooden skeletons are vulnerable in some way to fire damage, or any kinds of fire-based attacks.

Behaviors: Wooden Skeletons do not feel fear and will not run away. They will attack the nearest humanoid, but will not attack plants or animals.

Number of Enemies: There should be at least one enemy per player character so that each player character can potentially "destroy" one enemy. If it does not make the battle too difficult, having two or three enemies more than the number of players may be worthwhile.

Supporting Growth

Core Capacity—Planning

In many strategy-based TTRPGs, combat can provide exciting opportunities for players to use their characters' abilities to develop tactical responses to a challenge. In this encounter, because the skeletons are made of wood, the players can think logically about their most effective attacks (or with some assistance from a GM). For example, encouraging players who use fire in their attacks against the wooden skeletons will show them the power of creative thinking and understanding their character's abilities. It is always important to reward creative approaches, but combat is the perfect place to help make it clear that logical and well thought out choices can have more opportunity for success, and a greater (or more spectacular) result.

Encounter 04: Frozen Vines

The party discovers a hidden cave, but frozen vines block the cave entrance.

Encounter Type: Exploration
Encounter Tone: Lighthearted
Core Capacities: Planning, Collaboration

Read-Aloud Script

"As you travel deeper into the Viney Woods you can feel the air getting colder and colder. The chill feels unnatural, like it is cutting straight through your clothes and into your bones.

It takes you some time to find the cave entrance that Kitcha told you about, but after some wandering about you are able to track it down.

The cave entrance is just as Kitcha described, with vines grown completely around it, creating an impassable barrier. However, it has also frozen over, you can see icicles hanging down from various points along the vines. It isn't hard to identify that the vines are hard as rock, too.

How are you going to get through this mess to the cave inside?"

Game Master Summary

The vines cover the entrance to the cave, and they are also frozen over, making them hard as rock. This is another quantum quandary, and can be solved by any number of approaches.

Respond to the player's suggestions, but make sure that no one suggestion or action by a single player is enough to solve the whole problem. Instead, the suggestions from the players should each make small progress, letting them all contribute to the solution together.

You have control over the world, so if you need to have the vines and ice react to the player's ideas to slow them down, have them re-grow or become stronger. Similarly, you can have them be destroyed through any suggestion that helps you move forward. The choice is yours.

Read the "So Then" text when the vines are destroyed and the player characters are able to pass into the cave.

Desire: Enter the cave.

Obstacle: Frozen vines cover the cave entrance.

Tactic: Destroy the vines, thaw the vines, or find another way inside.

So Then: *"As you step into the cave you can smell the horrible stench of death. It is clear that you must be on the right track, though what awaits you further in, you cannot know."*

Game Master Notes

Some players love exploration challenges like these, with plenty of opportunity to explore and plenty of time to do it in. However, other players need more of a push and are more engaged in a game that has higher stakes. Remember that the important part of this encounter is to provide collaborative problem solving from the players, and having them fully engaged and interested may significantly improve their willingness to collaborate. You can change this encounter in any way that you see fit, and the only thing needed to keep the story on track is to make it through the wall (or defeat it) and into the cave at the end. As the GM, you can change the game to be the most engaging that it can be for the players at your table.

One option may be to have the frozen vines lash out against the player characters, pulling them in and threatening to freeze the characters to the Viney wall. Another might be to have the frozen vines grow rock-like thorns which they can explode toward anyone they meet. You can even bring back more wooden skeletons (if your players had fun fighting them before).

Lastly, perhaps as a GM you're simply short on time and need to bring this story to a close. You can always let the first suggestion be successful in getting through the vines, allowing you to progress further through the story, or skip this encounter entirely.

Supporting Growth

Core Capacity—Collaboration

Reinforcing collaboration, especially in a quantum quandary, is about finding any opportunity to show that ideas working together are far more effective and impactful than individual ideas. Reward players who come up with plans together, or who suggest ideas that assist the suggestion of another player, by making those far more likely to be successful and more spectacular in their success. Use the descriptive nature of the game to add more expansive and exciting descriptive words to their suggestions. It is alright to make these things more clear to the player, when needed, as well. For example, you could say "That might be tough to do, you'd probably be more successful if someone wanted to help you out in some way." Or, "Your character knows that would be challenging to accomplish on their own, what do they say to their teammates to ask for help?" Making it clear that player characters can talk to each other, can ask each other for help or make suggestions in character, can help to remind players that success in this game, and in many other places, depends on good teamwork and relationships with others.

Encounter 05: Burial Rites

The heroes must quell Eera's ghost to perform the burial incantation and put her to rest.

Encounter Type: Combat or Social
Encounter Tone: Serious
Core Capacities: Collaboration, Pretend Play

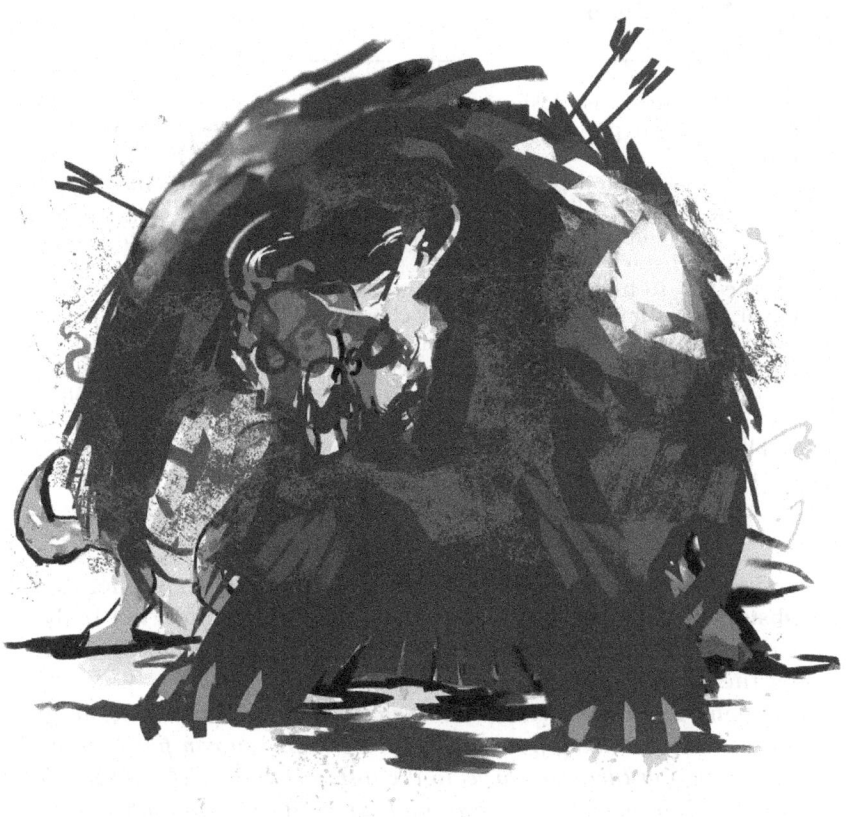

Figure 15.2 Eera the Owlbear

Read-Aloud Script

"The cave is not as deep as you might assume. It is only a turn around the corner before you are faced with what you seek.

You can see that there is a large open section to the cave, like the size of a den or great room. Toward the center back of the cave is the body of an owlbear, long dead. Several swords and javelins, rusted and rotted with time, protrude from the corpse.

Before you have a chance to move toward it, you can hear a screeching howl, a sound filled with fear and pain, coming from behind you. Eera clearly does not appreciate you setting foot in this place.

A spectral form of a bear, covered in feathers, with an owl-like face and beak appears, cutting off your exit, and charges toward you! (Figure 15.2) Eera attacks!"

Game Master Summary

This encounter is designed as a boss encounter, but with the flexibility that players can creatively negotiate their way through it if needed.

Eera is designed to be more interesting and more challenging than the Wooden Skeletons from earlier. She should represent a significant challenge for the players who are interested in having a harder obstacle.

One way to help this fight feel more challenging is to make sure that Eera inflicts damage to every character. It is also a good idea to keep track of character's hit points so that you can intentionally get a player character close to death without crossing over that line.

If the players want to chat or negotiate with Eera, you can follow the instructions in the Eera role-play pop-out block on the next page.

This encounter ends when the players defeat Eera through combat or through role-play.

Desire: Enact the burial incantation on Eera's body to put her to rest.
Obstacle: Eera's ghost will attack the heroes and protect her body.
Tactic: Subdue Eera's spirit with physical or magical attacks, or show her the intent to bring her peace.
So Then: *"As Eera's spirit vanishes you can hear an almost relief or appreciative whistle coming from the wind. Perhaps you can finally help this spirit rest. You turn your focus to the task at hand, ready to help Eera's body finally be placed into the ground, where it can help contribute to the cycle of nature as it should."*

Game Master Notes

GMs should make the choice of combat versus role-play based on the needs and choices of the players in the group. While some GMs may prefer one choice over the other, the player character's actions should be what dictate the best route.

Remember that it is a collaborative story, and the players will feel more heard and a stronger sense of contribution to the story if you let them make a choice which impacts the results.

Role-playing Eera

The player characters can attempt to talk Eera out of her blind vengeance and hate, but must put themselves at risk to do so.

Eera seeks release from her torment and wants what the player characters are offering, a chance to bury her body and let her rest. She simply doesn't understand that the player characters are here to perform that task, and instead thinks they are here to further desecrate what was once her home.

If the players want to show that they are not there as a threat to Eera, you can have them roll checks for what they know about animals or owlbears for the best ways to show that they are not a threat. Provide clear answers for the players to follow such as they can put down their weapons or hold up their hands.

You do not have to have Eera speak, instead describing her actions and body language to the players, along with an interpretation of the meaning. Even if you're acting out Eera's body language, you may need to give explicit meaning or words to that body language for the players to understand.

The Spirit of Eera

Eera is intended to be a spirit, or ghost-like being. GMs should select a monster or beast from their game to be appropriate for the level of their players. Adding in special qualities related to being a spirit will help make the battle more exciting and immersive.

Special Qualities: Spirit Form: Eera is a vengeful spirit, and cannot be bound. Physical attacks affect her, but any attempt to bind her with physical objects (vines, ropes, etc.) does not work. She can pass right through them. Magical attempts to bind Eera also do not work. She is immune to all forms of paralysis.

Behaviors: Eera will attack the nearest player to her, but will stop attacking if the players attempt to show that they are not a threat.

Number of Enemies: Eera is the only enemy in this battle, but if you feel like the players need more challenge (or more targets), you can add one to two wooden skeletons. Be careful not to make the battle too challenging for the players, they should still win.

Supporting Growth

Core Capacities—Perspective

Some groups will benefit from having an overt "bad guy" and a clear objective without the need to navigate moral difficulties. Others may benefit from having Eera present as a sympathetic character who needs compassion, not combat. Eera can be played specifically as a tragic figure, providing opportunity for players to better understand their perspective. You can adjust the difficulty of this challenge by changing the kind of communication that Eera uses, such as having Eera only communicate with noises and body language (as an animal might) rather than using words.

Encounter 06: Epilogue

The heroes have successfully laid Eera to rest.

Read-Aloud Script

> *"With the forest spirit at ease, you spend some time following Kitcha's instructions. Once the body is buried and a burial rite is said, you can finally make your way back to Wandershore.*
> *By the time you make your way back to Wandershore it is well into the evening and you expect a sleepy little town like this to be quiet and still. Instead you find the town of Wandershore to be in a celebratory uproar. It would appear that breaking the curse also freed the missing townspeople, who immediately found their way back to town.*
> *You're immediately overwhelmed with appreciation and applause for your efforts. The town is heralding you as heroes and they offer you food and songs through the night in celebration. You're also offered a comfortable bed and place to stay for as long as you should wish.*
> *Tensa pays you the money that she owes you, and several townspeople kick in their own money in appreciation, paying you each an extra 5 gold pieces."*

Game Master Notes

This encounter is designed to provide player input into the conclusion of the story. There are no DOTS for this encounter, as it is generally focused on collaborative world building.

The GM should lead the players through the conclusion of the story, and the results of their heroism. The storyline results should contain and wrap up important loose ends that had been established in the story, including having the missing townsfolk reappear from the woods. However, this is also a good opportunity to invite the players to be a part of the storytelling more directly.

The questions listed in the following are only a guide for the GM, you do not need to ask any of them, and it is not recommended to ask all of them. The goal of this encounter is to have fun collaborating on the end of the story and, if needed, into a new mystery that the players can pursue after this one. Some of the questions listed are intentionally open ended, providing a lot of opportunity for player input, and some are intentionally closed, providing only a small selection of choices available. Some players do well with open-ended questions, while others do well with more closed-ended ones. Use your knowledge of the players to choose the best options for each of them.

Collaborative Story Questions:

- What does the celebration of your return look like?
- What kind of food do they have at the celebration?
- The townspeople set up some decorations once they saw that the curse had been lifted. What color are the decorations?
- This town has activities that they like to do during celebrations, such as dancing or playing games. What kind of activity do they do?
- Tensa, the town elder, gives you each a small, but meaningful, hand carved figurine. What does your character's figurine look like?
- Tensa has a gift for telling fortunes and provides each of your characters a free fortune telling. What does she tell your character about their future?
- How does your character participate in the celebrations?

As the GM you can also role-play the interactions with the townspeople, or use the description in the read-aloud text to conclude the story. You can also use this as an opportunity to launch into a new story. The player characters can move on to visit a new town and discover a new opportunity for adventure, or you can prompt a new story direction for them by having a messenger—perhaps one who heard of their triumph in the Viney Woods—show up with a plea for their help.

Supporting Growth

Core Capacity—Collaboration

Encounters like this one, focused on player-based collaborative storytelling, have wonderful opportunities to build on each other's ideas. Remember that your body language and engagement with players are significant tools in your arsenal for growth. As the facilitator and GM you command and control the room, and the players pay close attention to you. You can use your presence to help encourage the player's attention along with you. Reward players who build on the ideas of others using your excitement and affect. You can also customize the questions to make it clear that players can build on each other's ideas. Such as asking a second player a follow-up question based on the first player's original answer.

Index

Note: Page numbers in *italics* indicate a figure, and page numbers in **bold** indicate a table on the corresponding page.

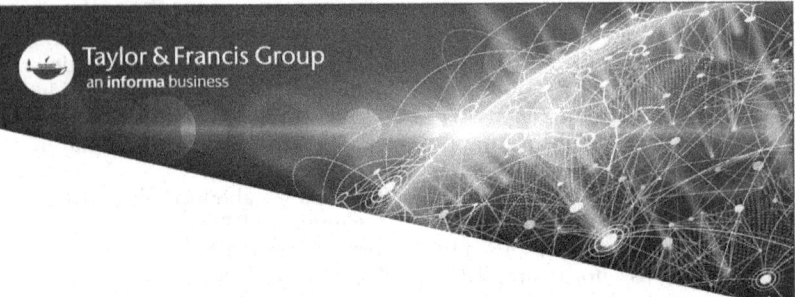
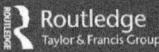
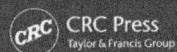